Till the Fat Lady Slims 2.0

The 'When Diet'

including

Exclusive Bonus Material

By Debbie Flint

Published by flintproductions

First published worldwide in hardback and e-Edition – 2015

QVC V1

hardback – ISBN - 978-1-909785-37-3
if available –
eBook – ISBN 978-1-909785-39-7
paperback – ISBN 978-1-909785-38-0

Amazing front cover illustration by Angela Oltmann
www.angieocreations.com

Caricature: Jef Thornton

Originally published by Sahara Publications

Published by Flintproductions

www.debbieflint.com @debbieflint

Till the
Fat Lady Slims
2.0

The 'When Diet'

including

Bonus Material

By Debbie Flint

Incorporating the original 2002 version plus additional bonus material for 2015

Dedication: with the utmost gratitude and big hugs to all the lovely friends and relations and Freedom Eaters out there who have all made this such a 'must-have' on their weight loss journey. For all the fabulous new testimonials since the QVC 'Back to You' show began in 2014, when people began asking how I'd been losing weight again. May your curiosity continue to repay you. Thanks to you all.

And to all my new readers, and regulars on my @qvcuk blog on www.qvcuk.com, I thank you all for taking the plunge and ordering this book. I await your feedback with anticipation!

I'D LOVE YOUR THOUGHTS

I'd really appreciate a review on Amazon or Goodreads! Or just email me on debbie@debbieflint.com. Enjoy!

Keeping in touch -

Go to www.debbieflint.com where you can -

- Sign up for updates and get my regular newsletter
- Plus news of free downloads and short stories
- A full list of my novels
- Follow my weekly well being blog
- Find *RiWiSi* – Read It Write It Sell It – my weekly look at all things book.
- And importantly, BONUS MATERIAL exclusive to readers of this book.

Or keep in touch via

Twitter @debbieflint

Or Facebook - search DebbieFlintQVC

Or Goodreads.

Table of Contents

About The Author, pre-2002 8

About the Author – 2014 9

Testimonials 11

PART ONE 16

The 'Super Six' – the Basic Principles of Freedom Eating 17

How to Incorporate The 'When' Diet into Any Diet Plan. 22

What if my body just can't have certain foods? 24

Tips on Sticking with the Programme 28

Whilst I was Away... BONUS MATERIAL - EXCLUSIVE 31

What Happened Next? 2000 - 2002 33

Now, Winter 2014 - What do I do? 43

PART TWO – Further Resources & the 'DF Plan!' 45

a. Sugar Prison 45

a. A Word about Fat v Sugar 47

b. Omega 3 Fish Oils 48

What do I do? The 'DF Plan' 51

Research and Further Reading 2014 53

PART THREE – 54

(TTFLS 2002 Original version) 54

TILL THE FAT LADY SLIMS (2002) - abridged 55

This was me in 1999..55

Where it all Began c.1999...59

About The Author c.2001 60

Enter the Fat Lady..61

The secret food prisoner 63

Chapter One – In the World of the Fat 65

Chapter Two –In the World of the Slim 73

Chapter Three - Ten Pounds of Lard......................................77

Chapter Four - Do What I Do 82

Chapter Five - Suffering the Slings and Arrows 86

Chapter Six - A Partner in Crime 93

Chapter Seven - Ecstasy on a Plate.......................................98

Chapter Eight - Hunger Know Thyself..................................103

Chapter Nine - What 'They' Say...106

Chapter Ten - More From the Fat Lady 111

Chapter Eleven - Emotional Eating 121

Chapter Twelve - This Whole Identity Thing 126

Chapter Thirteen - Food Freedom in a Nutshell....................134

Chapter Fourteen - Binge Management 150

The Key Points to Food Freedom 169

Testimonials - 1999 - 2002 170

Appendix - References 173

Further reading & Support Groups Online 174

Bonus Material 175

incl Debbie's Fiction, and Keeping in Touch

About The Author, pre-2002

At the time of writing the original book, Debbie Flint was at QVC the Shopping Channel, first time round. Previously, she had trained as an accountant, and took a business degree at the London School of Economics before entering the world of TV and Radio. Having started her broadcasting career in radio, she became the first female presenter in the Children's BBC Broom Cupboard. That was followed by marriage, the arrival of her two children, stints on BBC Daytime TV, Living TV and ten years with Children's SSVC TV Forces' Television. In 1998, Debbie returned to BBC1 to host her own game show Meet the Challenge. However, Debbie is probably best known from her work on UK Shopping Television - including QVC from 1994. There, in 1999, she came across the book and tape pack from Vikki Hansen and Shawn Goodman about the method of natural weight loss called **Freedom Eating**. Having used it herself to great effect, and due to viewers' requests, Vikki and Shawn asked her to write her own version, which was then picked up by Sahara Publications Limited for the 2002 original 'Till the Fat Lady Slims.'

In 2000, Debbie said, "In all my years of seeing thousands of products on Shopping TV, none had as much impact on me as the **Freedom Eating** pack - it may sound clichéd but it's literally changed my life. Vikki and Shawn the creators, will eternally be in my heart as the ladies who helped me break free from Food Prison for the first time! Without them, the last few years of troubles ('99-'01) would have led to a massive weight gain. (*Ed. The original was finished around the time Debbie was getting divorced.)* Instead of that, despite all the traumas, I've managed to stop bingeing forever – and lose 2 stone!" Debbie says.

In this original comprehensive guide to **Food Freedom**, as Debbie referred to it, she added her own spin, and shared some of the most intimate secrets of her dieting diary. How this system can be combined with a traditional diet, and the introduction of **Binge Management**. So, in an attempt to explain **Freedom Eating** further, and in order to bring it up to date with her original experience, she tells her own story. **Freedom Eating** gets a personalised twist.

About the Author – 2014

Nowadays, Debbie Flint is divorced and lives In Dorking with her three Labradors and her two children, Lauren and Bradley are happily settled with their partners. As of 2009, she is back doing the job she loves – a TV presenter on QVC the Shopping Channel. She also writes steamy romance novels which she self-publishes on Amazon etc, and in summer 2014 signed a publishing deal for her Hawaiian trilogy with Choc Lit, the innovative independent UK publisher.

Twelve years after the original 'Till the Fat Lady Slims' (TTFLS) was published, Debbie was asked to write an update. With the advent of Debbie's well-being show, 'Back to You,' on QVC – a whole new generation began using Freedom Eating to lose weight and change their habits around food. But since the world has moved on since 2002, this version now incorporates new thinking about how to use her system alongside traditional methods. Plus some fabulous bonuses.

In this new 2015 update you will find these extras –

- the 'When' Diet – the basic principles of Freedom Eating, in a nutshell. 'The Super Six' – the eating habits of a slim person. How to use them alongside ANY traditional diet. Crucial for those who cannot let go of structured methods of weight loss.
- advice about the dangers of sugar addiction – extra resources to help you escape the fructose trap so you can trust your body's signals
- brand new testimonials, including Chloe, 25, who has lost four stone between January and September 2014, and many more
- links to extra info & podcast/audiobook
- **PLUS - Bonus material exclusive to this edition** –
- Debbie's story, 2002 – 2014, *in-depth*
- *exclusive* one month routine for beginners - **The 'DF Plan!'**

Baby Steps

This book is designed to be read, and re-read, on a regular basis to help you adjust to the new patterns of behaviour. Please note the changes will take time, for most people.

Disclaimer

Please note - this book attempts to provide guidance for the understanding of natural eating. It is not, in any way, shape or form, a medical manual or a guide to treatment. If you think you may have a medical problem, you must see your medical practitioner. Nutritional needs are different from one person to another, and from one situation to another, including differences in gender, age and general health. Therefore you must use this book as a means of helping you make informed decisions about your dietary regime. This book is not a substitute for any treatment prescribed by your doctor. In order to ensure the confidentiality of the people who have written to the author, many of the surnames have not been included.

The author of this book is not a medical professional. Her aim is not to dispense any medical advice, directly or indirectly, regarding any technique mentioned in this book. You must always check with your medical practitioner before you start on any regime mentioned or described in this book. The aim is to give you, the reader, general information, based on the author's own experience, to help you in your search for a slimmer, healthier body. The author, the editor and the publishers, therefore assume no responsibility for your actions in the event of the use of any of the information in this book.

Testimonials

Chloe Hillier, age 25 – lost 4 stone 24th September 2014

"I started my weight loss journey in January this year. I started using the freedom eating principles combined with exercise after reading Debbie's book TTFLS. The main thing that I am pleased about is how it's enabled me to have a healthy, positive relationship with food. If I overindulge... I'm not 'punishing' myself like I used to or experiencing the awful guilt that I used to put myself through. I was shocked to find out that I had even lost a pound whilst on holiday in Thailand for two weeks and I really did treat myself to lovely food! I have now lost four stone and recently treated myself to a size 12 dress :) previously I was wearing size 18-20! I will continue to use the freedom eating principles even when I reach my goal weight!"

Bev, TTFLS Facebook group 9th September 2014

"My pre-freedom eating clothes no longer fit. I used to be size 12 bottoms and 14 tops, now I'm size 8/10. Obviously I'm thrilled with my new shape but more importantly I feel more confident and balanced. Because I now control my food, not vice versa, and my eating is guilt free. Freedom eating is a way of life for me now, no more dieting or calorie counting. Just wholesome food and only when I'm truly hungry. I've lost at least 2 stone and gone down two dress sizes, effortlessly!"

Debbie Sinclair Bunn, TTFLS Facebook group. *11th September 2014*

"It's so liberating to NOT be on a diet, all I can say is one day at a time, listen to your body. Knowing when you need water rather than food is an amazing breakthrough, it took me a few weeks. Throwing out my scales was also a fantastic feeling ... the hardest bit I think is being honest with yourself. I have been a yo-yo dieter for years - been to clubs, had diet pills the lot, but TTFLS has finally worked for me ..."

Marcella, TTFLS Facebook group 7th September 2014

"Before reading Debbie's TTFLS...I'd always had a guilty relationship with food ever since I can remember - shouldn't eat this...shouldn't eat that...I won't have dinner because I feel fat and don't deserve it - then I'd binge on crisps and olives when the kids had gone to bed because I was ravenous!...and then I felt like a bloated failure!

I had tried lots of so called healthy eating plans but found them to be extremely boring...and so I would fall into my bad habits again. I never weigh myself but go by how certain items of clothing fit instead...and since 'listening' to the book, I have found that I can eat when I'm hungry...and not just for the sake of it...it can be done, will power is needed of course but I just keep thinking about what's in the book....I'm eating healthier too - cooking veg and eating salads instead of having chips for dinner every day - I also don't beat myself up any more, about having a take away meal every Wednesday after the kids have their swimming lessons... it's our little treat.

It was also great to find out that I wasn't the only one having a battle with food...and even better to find that there was someone willing and able to put it down in writing for those of us who need some guidance! Last year I was disappointed in myself because I couldn't fit into the dress I wanted to wear...then this August - a REAL smile because I could finally wear the dress!... Yayy!

It's funny because the book has helped me see that I can have freedom with other things too... how I feel about myself, how I dress... and how I deal with my children!! - Freedom - not to conform to how others think I should be - I just needed to be 'me'... and I'm starting to like myself again - it's been a very long time since I have been able to say that!... I even took the kids swimming on Wednesday after their lesson ended... I just put my tankini in the bag and off we went - I didn't worry about whether or not I had hair products, make-up, jewellery or anything!... and I survived!... haha... thanks for this great little book, Debbie, it's helped me to be me again!... xxxx"

Jill Dowding Walker – testimonial 6th September 2014

I am a middle-aged woman, married with one teenager. I also happen to be disabled with an illness that has impacted my mobility for many years, finally diagnosed in 2008. Being less and less able to move in the whirlwind fashion I previously enjoyed, now often confined to bed or wheelchair, my weight increased and my exercise lessened because it was too painful and exhausting. Inevitably I gained more and more weight.

In combination with a few other motivational tools, (and near starvation, feeling hungry all the time) I did manage to reduce my weight by three and a half stones within a year. Unfortunately as I lost interest for a period, I regained five stones over the next two years! Then I found TTFLS and the simple, clear advice resonated with me.

Reading TTFLS was an eye-opener! Written in a friendly tone and supportive manner, it helped me realise I was far from alone in my struggles with food...

I now recognise when I am hungry and when I am not. You would think that was simple, but it takes time to build habits and interpret the signals from your body to ascertain this. TTFLS explains why and how to learn strategies to overcome this disconnection, or misunderstanding the language of your body.

My top tips were learning to recognise what I wanted and when I really wanted it, whatever time of day, or situation I was in. I learned to question myself. What was I feeling? What did my body need? Was I sufficiently hydrated? So, was I thirsty or really hungry?

Also, when I am eating, no matter what, or how hungry I am, as soon as I notice myself taking a breath and sighing, I know it is a signal to stop eating now. Why do we sigh? Usually and unconsciously it is because our body is satisfied.

There are many more tips in Debbie's book, but those above are especially the ones that have positively impacted my eating habits..."

INTRODUCTION

Winter 2014

This updated book is in three parts. My 2002 original version is still included – even twelve years later its message still holds, and has been helping a lot of people overcome their lifelong battle with weight gain and to start leading a normal life around food. I've heard from so many who tell me not only are they losing weight but are becoming happier within themselves.

I learned the Freedom Eating system in 1999, when it helped me lose 35lb, quit binge eating, and mostly keep it off over the next decade and a half. In its entirety, you let go of deprivation and control and trust your body to choose the right thing in the right quantity at the right time. Everything changes when you let go of the reins. That original version is reproduced - abridged - at the end of this book. Nothing else has ever worked for me the way the complete Freedom system does.

BUT not everybody can take that plunge and let go straight away. I heard from people who were incorporating elements of Freedom Eating to adapt their habits more gradually. I chatted to my sister Linda – a former slimming club leader – and she has helped me develop The 'When' Diet - the absolute fundamentals of my Freedom Eating system, to be used in conjunction with ANY traditional plan. If you're like Linda and prefer to work to a structured programme – this is for you. Whereas for me, you start telling me I can't eat something, it only makes me want it even more! Full Freedom Eating works for me. So there's something for everyone in this 2015 update.

Plus, given the current wave of findings about fructose and the health dangers of sugar, it needed a revamp to keep up with the times, since some people find it hard to listen to their body when it is addicted to sugar. I also added other pertinent info and resources.

In addition, this book contains brand new 2014 testimonials from my new 'Till the Fat Lady Slims' Facebook group. You are welcome to join – it's a great support system. You'll find links to that and other superb resources to help you in your journey. On my website, www.debbieflint.com you'll find the latest before and after stories too.

Finally, this limited edition contains special exclusive Bonus Material. I've dug deep into my memories to share with you one of the most difficult times of my life and how I got through it, finally embracing Freedom Eating again to return to my ideal weight.

Enjoy the book, and commence your own journey. When you're ready. And don't forget to leave me that all important review at the end!

Best wishes

Debs

x

30th August 2014 - Lynne Sneddon – TTFLS Facebook group

"My family and my Mum went to the Harvester last night to celebrate our 12th wedding anniversary (today) and my Mum's birthday on Monday and I have to say I am rather impressed with myself. I visited the salad bar and didn't have any dressing or anything like croutons or crispy onions on my salad bowl. For my main course I chose the gammon steak with peas and jacket potato with no butter. For sweet, I had fruit salad with vanilla ice cream. The ice cream was served in a tiny cup similar to an expresso cup. Drink wise I went for diet cola as I didn't fancy any alcohol. We had a fab time and I thoroughly enjoyed my meal. I could have chosen a huge rhubarb & custard sundae or a honeycomb one like my mom but I didn't feel hungry enough to know that I would have enjoyed it but I wanted something sweet to finish my meal off. The fruit and ice cream did the trick without feeling full to bursting. #TTFLSisKickingIn – hopefully I will get slim in time to renew our wedding vows in the Canary Islands in 2 years' time"

PART ONE

FREEDOM EATING STAGE ONE – THE 'WHEN' DIET

By popular demand, I've now separated out the basic principles of Freedom Eating and called it 'The *'When'* Diet'. It's the foundation of Freedom Eating. If you are a beginner, this is where you start. It transforms your focus from a list of 'must nots' – of avoiding lots of foods – to place the emphasis instead onto a type of game. A game you play with yourself. You can't lose, or fail, or be wrong. You can only learn.

This is where you accurately pick the right time to eat, the right match for the food you need in that moment, and then observe what happens in your body afterwards. It's all about when rather than what. Remember – and this is alien to so many of us failed dieters – there's no 'wrong' – there's only learning, honing, and getting more accurate next time. And with this system 'next time' is a few hours later – at the very next meal time. Not 'tomorrow,' not 'on Monday.' And it's taking back the keys to your prison – your food prison.

Because it's time to break free.

The Basics of the When Diet.

I'm listing the basic principles of Freedom Eating here, right up front, so that you can get a snapshot of what this book is all about. The full in-depth explanation, along with what happened to me when I first discovered it all those years ago, is later in the book. But this is the nuts and bolts of what to do.

It's not magic, it's common sense – but for many of us, we stopped doing it a long time ago. The rest of this book will help you keep doing it.

Also please note Part Two - about sugar addiction – and spend time doing further research – since you can't trust a body that's addicted. This is all relatively new science. If you're like me, and hate dieting, counting stuff and being told 'you can't,' then stages one, two AND three – are a life-changer. But we'll start with stage one.

The 'Super Six' – the Basic Principles of Freedom Eating

1. **Wait till you're 6 on the hunger scale**, when the signals will be clearer to you about what your body genuinely wants to eat this mealtime. Think of it like the fuel light going on in your car. Only when you're sufficiently hungry will you make the right food choices. You're not saying 'I can't have that food – you're saying the opposite – I can have that food – WHEN the time is right.

2. **Be accurate in what you choose** – try to eat when you can have exactly what your body wants. Really listen to the signals your body is giving you as you consider each food choice. Ask yourself a series of questions if you're a beginner – do I want sweet or savoury, hot or cold, rich or bland, crunchy or creamy… etc. Then really imagine eating a food – the taste of it in your mouth – the sixth sense about how it will make you feel. Some people even smack their lips and close their eyes at this point. The food that 'shouts' the loudest to you is the right one in that moment.

   Tip 1 – if you can't tell what you need most, or *everything* is appealing, you're probably thirsty, so drink a big glass of water (the purer the better) and try again in 15 minutes.

   Tip 2 – it's OK to delay eating until later WHEN you can make sure you have exactly the right food choices to hand. Some go hungry a bit longer just to get the food choice spot-on, as the rewards are so great (see The Bliss Point game, in 7 below.) Meanwhile a little of something to fill the gap is OK, just try to make it as accurate as you can for your body's needs at that time.

   Tip 3 – if you're on a traditional 'diet plan,' this is where tdhe 'When' Diet clicks in – but you just make your choices from the list of foods on your plan. Simply be as accurate as you can even within the more confined range of foods on your plan.

3. **Pay full attention to your food**. Don't eat until a time WHEN you can do absolutely nothing else. If you're a beginner this means literally NOTHING else – don't talk, watch TV, read, or drive and definitely don't pick up the next forkful ready to

shove it in your mouth. Take your time – almost like doing a food meditation. Focus on the food and give it your full attention. If you're going to pick from the fridge at least pull up a chair! Best of all, sit at a table to eat your meal. Beginners can even take themselves off somewhere suitable to sit down undisturbed to eat their food, so you can pick up on the subtle signals your body is going to give you about when to stop. Chew each mouthful for a long time, enjoy every morsel. Some people utter ecstatic 'mmmm' noises so sometimes that's good to do in private! Hehe!

4. THE MOST IMPORTANT POINT OF ALL **Stop eating WHEN satisfied NOT when full**. As I said the first time I came across this alien concept – 'What, you mean you don't keep eating till you can't breathe anymore?!'

   This is probably the biggest change to your habits, and is absolutely VITAL. Once you do this, you can say you are Freedom Eating.

   Tip 1 – The point of satisfaction is most often indicated by your body taking a deep breath. It's a breath of relief. It's like your body is saying 'ahh, that's better, thank you, I'm done now.' But whilst hunger shouts, satisfaction WHISPERS – so it's vital to listen, observe, learn, and play The 'When' Diet game.
   Tip 2 – After the deep breath, the taste explosion may abate, your food flavour may seem to change and become less appealing. Your attention may also wander off the food.
   Tip 3 – It's likely to be after about a fist full of food: a SMALL plate full. Beginners - don't be surprised if it's half the amount you're used to.
   Tip 4 - It's OK to leave the rest – it really is. And it's OK to SAVE IT TILL LATER – till WHEN you are hungry enough all over again and it will taste just as good. Doggy bags or To-Go bags or a little plastic container with an airtight lid are worth using. Or put the food in the fridge covered up ready for later!
   Tip 5 – Beginners, be prepared for funny quips and comments from those around you, but don't try to argue or educate others – they may be food prisoners and haven't got the secret that you have. They are still conditioned but you are breaking free.

Tip 6 – This is a magic one – Just say 'I don't **feel** like it now but I'd love it later'. That usually works a treat. This is where social conditioning must be ignored and you can let go of the learned drive to finish your plate. No-one will mind. Remember, just say 'I don't **feel** like any more but I'd love to save it till later.' It all means you've had enough and can give yourself permission to stop now, in order to experience the next stage.

5. **Aim for the Bliss Point.** THEN play the Bliss Point game: be a detective and watch out for the moment your body rewards you for getting it exactly right. Your body will be filled with an overwhelming feeling of happiness and floaty satisfaction, and a quiet calm. It means you gave your body exactly what it needed that mealtime. Hooray! It's a freedom, a feeling of control, and it sets you up ready for the next meal time. Once you're used to it, nothing else will do. Foodies will adore Freedom Eating because you never eat unless it's WHEN the food tastes absolutely heavenly. Every. Single. Time. It's like some sort of pleasure ride. Stopping at the right time, having eaten at the right time, and only eating when you can consume the right foods, that's the 'When' Diet. And it feels exhilarating. You may even get a rush of joy, realising that this is how your whole life can be from now on. No more feeling guilty after a meal, or bad or sad.

   Tip 1 – If your choice doesn't achieve this, and the food just tasted kind of 'OK' then you probably didn't get it right this time. BUT don't worry, let it go. DO NOT BEAT YOURSELF UP if you overshot and ate a little too much this time. Just wait till you're hungry again later and begin the game again. Think – When is it time to eat? When will I be able to eat exactly what my body wants, and when am I satisfied? It's all about observation, rather than deprivation.

   Tip 2 – Also do not beat yourself up if you had something formerly 'bad' – eg, chocolate or some chips. Things that previously made you feel like you'd 'broken' your diet and made you feel a failure. With Freedom Eating there is no 'bad,' there's only 'inaccurate.' This is a different game you're playing now and as long as you're honest, and only eat between being hungry and being satisfied, and genuinely choosing what your body (not your brain) wants, then you're playing the beginner's When Diet game. You just have more to learn.

Tip 3 – No more 'treasure foods.' The more you do this, the tastier real food will be. You may notice how much less appealing all those 'naughty' foods are if you know they're not like treasure any more. You're a step nearer to getting it right more frequently and 'winning' the game. It's OK, for instance, if you eat what used to be 'treasure' foods – now you won't panic and and eat everything left in the cupboards. Wait till the next meal time and start the game all over again – if you've not gone past satisfied, it'll only be a few hours away. Most importantly do not beat yourself up, or think you've failed. And definitely don't punish yourself for 'breaking' your diet plan by eating ten times what your body actually wants. Those are old habits, and the 'When' Diet means you can't 'break' a diet, you're just playing a learning game. Learning to trust in your body again.

6. **Examine the way your body feels afterwards** and don't repeat the same choices next time if it made you feel bad. This is where you become your own science project. Even if you ended up deciding to consume cake or chips or crisps or whatever, it's important to do the When Diet and crucially stop when satisfied. Then listen to your body some more – listen anew to the signals in your body.

   It's a game, it's an experiment, and you are the scientist, conducting 'choice and timing experiments' on your own body in a way that will change your life forever. There is no failure at this game, there are only more-accurate and less-accurate timing and food choices.

   As long as you eat within the above principles, you can combine *Freedom Eating (Stage One): the When Diet*, with absolutely ANY diet plan out there. ANY.

   That is the basic premise of this book. If you have read enough and think you know all that, you don't need to read on. If however, this is a revelation, as it all was to me in 1999, then read it several times. Many people don't 'get it' straight away - take baby steps, gradually adopting the principles above into your life. If you've been getting it wrong for a long, long time, it may feel alien but it will happen – trust your body, it's a wonderful thing. (& see TTFLS original, in Part Three.)

27th September – Cath Purple – TTFLS Facebook group

"When I was born, some foods were still being rationed and it was hard to get certain items. Consequently I was indeed brought up to eat everything that was put on my plate! I remember food from a previous meal being given to me at the next meal and the next until I had eaten it! Mealtimes seemed to be a constant battle. This has stuck with me for the whole of my life and I have often struggled to complete a plateful if food, in order not to leave any.

What a liberating book is TTFLS! Suddenly I have been 'given permission' to leave food if I don't want it - not because I don't like it, but because I have had enough. I also now listen to my body and eat when I am hungry and not at set times! This new found liberation has had a knock on effect, because I am slowly feeling happy with myself and accepting that I am who I am. TTFLS is motivating in so many ways and I am feeling the shackles of the past melt away! Thank you Debbie Flint! Xx"

How to Incorporate The 'When' Diet into Any Diet Plan.

The 'When' Diet principles, incorporating the 'Super Six' above, can be used alongside any calorie-counting, points-counting, fasting or food restricting diet plan. You'll just have a narrower list of foods to choose from.

So – when you get to Principle 2, just choose what you feel like most from the food choices on your diet plan. You can still choose what shouts loudest to your body – do it as best you can, where possible.

And if it's not possible as your plan is a defined list of meals you eat on specific days, and you can't vary it, you can still do the rest of the principles – as follows –

1 – wait till you're 6 on the hunger scale

(2 – be accurate in what you choose: what's the best fit, right now?)

3 – pay full attention to your food, do nothing else whilst eating

4 – stop when you're satisfied. Listen to your body and stop WHEN it's time. If a diet instructs you to *'fill up* on fruits or vegetables', don't. No-one should 'fill up' – everyone should stop when satisfied – otherwise you're eating more than your body needs and it will get stored instead of used up.

5 – play the Bliss Game – assuming you have some degree of freedom. If not, just ensure you do Principles 1, 3, 4 and 6.

6 – this final principle is the most vital if you're on a diet which requires restriction, deprivation and control – do NOT beat yourself up if you come off it. Observe your body afterwards to help future choices.

BONUS - Diet-Rescue Plan

In fact, if you feel a binge coming on, check out 'binge management' later in this book.

And if you've 'broken' the diet, use Freedom Eating as a fall-back –

- Don't panic, don't beat yourself up, don't 'start again tomorrow' (principle 6)

- Do nothing – it's ok to just wait till you're hungry again (principle 1)

- If it works for you, analyse what happened and why you 'broke' your diet – it's all part of the learning process (principle 6)

- Just aim to begin again at principle number 1 and wait till the moment arrives and your body's ready to eat again. It may be a longer time to wait if you overate last time.

- Choose what your body really wants – even if it's from a more restricted list of options. And if being forced to choose from a restricted list is your trigger to panic again, then just choose from a wider range of healthier foods, if you have them to hand. If you don't, go get them. Give your body every chance to achieve a bliss point by picking exactly the right food (principle 5)

- When you're a little more comfortable again, drink some water.

- Don't have a Last Supper, just do Principle 2 and pick more freely from all the foods available to you.

- Stop when satisfied (principle 4)

- Revert to the 'When' Diet and know that you now have full freedom to choose, as long as you stop when satisfied. That knowledge alone may take the edge off your panic and tendency to disobey your specialist's 'diet' plan.

- Do the Super Six and get back on track with your 'diet' once the crisis has passed.

What if my body just can't have certain foods?

One final note. It concerns Principle 6. And here is where all the new information comes into operation. Information that wasn't around when I created the first Till the Fat Lady Slims in 2002.

You see, whilst you're learning to recognise your body's subtle signals about how to eat like a slim person all over again, certain knowledge may help you on your way. And it all hinges on Principle 6 of the Super Six.

Read on for –

- Help with recognising addiction
- Using research as an ally
- Tips on sticking with the programme
- Doctor's orders – using The 'When' Diet as a safety zone

If you 'need' to avoid any particular food, the chances are that if you eat it, your body will feel bad in some way.

Assuming that's the case, you may be amongst the group of people who react favourably to news and information. It helps you interpret your body's signals more clearly to stay on track.

I made a major breakthrough with my own body's needs when I discovered via a week-long cookery workshop that my body doesn't like dairy. And sugar actually gives me hangover symptoms. And meat slows down my system. That's my situation, it may or may not be yours. You may have other specific dietary needs. So I choose more wisely now I know.

What is your situation?

Everyone's will be unique to them.

The whole point about The 'When' Diet is that you can follow what works for you – only you know, based on how your body reacts.

But you have to learn to trust your body once again.

Recognising Addiction

But what if you can't trust it yet? If you're finding it difficult to stop yourself eating rubbish, eg you keep 'wanting' chocolate, your body may be throwing you a curve ball. The 'When' Diet Principle 6, means observe your body afterwards - maybe you're addicted to sugar.

That's where the new information comes in. There's so much now readily available online, or from an expert, or in newspapers and magazines. Filling your head with the right information can affect how you interpret your body's signals and the subsequent choices you make. Just like finding out that some sausages may be made with pigs lips, tails or trotters means some people never feel like eating sausages again, certain information in our heads, can affect our body's desires for some foods.

Sugar is a problem all on its own, however, as it's been called seven times more addictive than cocaine according to some studies (FABResearch.org) That's why I've included a whole new section about it below.

Ordinary table sugar is made up of half glucose and half fructose, and it's fructose, from fruit sugars, which is the problem. This is all new information, and has changed how I view the body's signals, because a body addicted to sugar will just keep demanding more sugar and the whole Freedom Eating process is hampered.

I advise giving it up – becoming un-addicted – and then you can more accurately read what your body is saying. After all, logically, we all know that no one should consume jelly babies and ice cream, milk chocolate and cake at every meal. But a lady in a sweet shop tried to do Freedom Eating by continually selecting from the huge range of candies at her fingertips and then couldn't understand why it didn't seem to be working. Another lady declared she was doing Freedom Eating and described how she'd gone and bought what she really fancied from the supermarket – a whole stack of cakes and biscuits – and slowly devoured most of them in the course of a day.

That's not Freedom Eating at work, that's sugar addiction.

So I offer you here a bit of extra research to help you work your way more accurately through the 6th Principle of the 'When' Diet.

Using Research as an Ally. For some, knowing more about the body makes a big difference. I changed my own interpretation of my body's signals when I found out what fructose does in the liver (from a Uni professor's YouTube video), and when I learned how a third of all the fructose calories we eat is automatically made back into fat (yes, really!). No matter what exercise you do nor what deficit you have – all calories really aren't the same.

Plus it also taught me how fruit juice can be VERY fattening (I'd been drinking a famous brand 'with bits' every day, slowly putting on weight and unable to think why - thinking juice was good for me. How wrong THAT was!) Also from 'food cure' expert Marlene Watson Tara, I discovered how simple carbohydrates (including chips, crisps, etc) also act like sugars and create insulin swings that actually prevent my body from releasing fat – whilst insulin is in your system it simply cannot get in the fat burning zone. In addition, new findings prove that the brain reacts to sugar the same way it reacts to cocaine or opiates: we really are addicted. It all makes me want to step in and refuse to let it control me.

Rather, I want to take back the power and be in control of me.

This kind of knowledge helps battle against addiction intellectually – and helps you understand better how to fight back against insidious, unnatural, man-made ingredients which will grab a hold of you before you know it. In my case, a little of what I fancy does NOT do me good. Particularly dairy.

I knew my body didn't like dairy – I used to bloat up something chronic and have asthma after I ate it. But via internet research, finding out that nearly two thirds of modern humans, globally, have lactose intolerance made me be able to say goodbye to it more easily. And I was someone who previously declared, 'no way ever would I want to give up cheese.' But feeling healthy is so, so much better than eating cheese. I also found out via Marlene Watson Tara (.com) and her macrobiotic courses that a plant-based, wholefood diet is the best thing for modern humans to eat in order to shed chronic illness and recover naturally.

Marlene took her brother's prostate cancer measurement down to a fraction of what it was, following a purely vegan diet along with miso soups, seaweeds, home-remedies like ginger compresses etc. Food is a medicine, or food is a poison – and it pays to know which is which.

There's a wealth of info out there, like never before. Watch the Youtube video 'Forks over Knives' for instance, and make your own mind up.

And it's not good enough anymore to remain ignorant of the glaring info that's come to light over the last decade. I saw a food programme where the mother said something like, 'Who'd have ever thought that by stopping little Harry having fizzy drinks every lunchtime and no more burger and chips and sweets, that it would have improved his behaviour so much. I had no idea what he ate was so connected to how he acted.'

I'm not saying the same techniques work for everyone – everybody's got a different story. But if the basics of Freedom Eating: the 'When' Diet - are taking a while to kick in for you, that's when it's time to 'go Google'. I'm urging you to go discover what your own story is.

23rd September - Elizabeth Grey – TTFLS Facebook group

"Well I've followed the mantra 'eat what I want when I want but only when I'm hungry' for the last 2 weeks. But no exercise other than the usual walk the dog. In a rush this morning pulled out a pair of trousers from wardrobe in semi darkness put them on not thinking and when I went downstairs realised I had not worn these trousers for 2 years because they didn't fit!! Well they do now and they are not elasticated waists or stretch - have proper waistband and zip so really pleased!..."

Tips on Sticking with the Programme

I know what to do, so how do I continuously 'Do What I Know?'

Look, we're all human. Even with all our knowledge, we still sometimes do stuff that's not best for us, don't we? It's only this year when Freedom Eating became my priority again – my fall back, my rescue plan – that I've lost the weight easily. Really easily, actually.

You see, doing all this research opened my eyes to 'food as medicine.' So when I got to principle 6 of the Super Six, and really thought about the effect of certain foods on my health, I found that it was just easier not to put my body through it. So it became easier to choose more wisely.

I know, by observing my body post-food, which foods I can have a bit of, and which I am just better off avoiding. Why give myself asthma by eating soft cheese, or custard or a latte with normal milk? For you, you may find once you're paying attention that you notice a certain brand of bread doesn't feel so good for you. Or eggs give you constipation. Or the kids play together much more calmly when they don't have certain ready meals, or half a can of soup containing four spoonfuls of sugar.

And through it all, you do it YOUR way...

My own way is that I'm not telling myself 'I can't.' I'm saying 'I can,' which changes the psychology. It means a food is not forbidden treasure, which means I consider whether I really WANT to eat it. And with all this new found knowledge, the answer is usually no, I don't.

So, so many things are possible.

And if all this seems alien to you, open your mind and your heart – because maybe, just maybe, you *'don't KNOW you don't know.'* An ex once said to me annoyingly, 'you can't help being ill,' just because he'd never come across the info I kept trying to tell him. He promptly kept eating cheese on white bread with thick butter, milky lattes, and staying at his brother's to look after the cats, then coming down with asthma attacks. Turns out he can't eat dairy either and is allergic to cats. *No Sh*t Sherlock!* Just because you've never heard of it – yet – doesn't mean it's not true. That's the reply to use, for many so-called health 'experts' who just haven't kept abreast of new findings.

There's too much info out there nowadays to remain ignorant of it all. Especially if you want to seriously take charge of your life. That's what it's been about for me – getting healthy as I hit 50 and making sure my next decades are energetic and free from aches and ailments. If you don't make time to be healthy now, you'll have to take time to be ill later. And I'm damn sure I don't want to spend my later decades being ill. Be your own science project, and do your research thoroughly, in order to wise up to what your body REALLY wants and what you're best off eating. And whenever you're feeling stressed or under pressure, go back to the Freedom Eating basics, because the 'When' Diet principles can help you battle through the difficult first few weeks of any 'giving up' procedure too.

Footnote - Doctors Orders – The 'When' Diet as a Safety Zone

If your diet means you HAVE to avoid certain foods, what do you do? Karen on Facebook asked me that, and my answer is – do all you can to stick to the advice of your professional.

BUT IF YOU CAN'T, IF IT DRIVES YOU MAD AND YOU CAN'T STAND IT, AND IF YOU FREQUENTLY BREAK THAT DIET and you know you shouldn't, that's where Freedom Eating kicks in as a safety zone.

Use it as a fall-back to help you make choices that will stop you going crazy. But do it **if - and only if -** it means you will avoid having a binge and feeling terrible, creating a vicious circle.

- Use it as a fall-back if it helps to minimize the time spent 'off the wagon.'

- Use it as a fall-back if the bliss point Freedom Eating gives you means you can avoid feeling bad about yourself

- Use it if it means you can get back on the straight and narrow pretty quickly afterwards.

If you're like me, the mere knowledge that you CAN have something means it's robbed of its 'treasure status' and you don't eat it after all. Freedom Eating is a safety zone – helping you stick to your prescribed 'diet.' This is how those on restricted diets may find Freedom Eating useful. (See also 'anatomy of a binge' later in this book.)

24th September – Chris Jopp – TTFLS Facebook Group

"When I first started reading Debbie Flint's book I didn't think it would have an impact on me but it did… it did leave an impression that's made me think about what I'm eating - and that's become so important to me.

The main thing I learned was that I don't need to think of myself as being on a diet! I am making better choices (most days LOL!) and although my weight loss is slow (by choice) I'm happy to go slowly. If I want to have something naughty, I have it but in a smaller portion and then I leave out something later in the day. If we eat out then hubby and I share a starter and/or a dessert (if we feel we want to have them) and if I want a starter or dessert to myself (I don't have both!) then I will cut out something from the main, like carbs. It's a process of substitution and portion control. And listening to your body.

Thank you Debbie, I'm re-reading it and look forward to the updated version. Xxxxx"

Whilst I was Away… BONUS MATERIAL - EXCLUSIVE

Most of the 'Till the Fat Lady Slims' original book – in Part Three of this updated version – is about full Freedom Eating, ie, following The 'When' Diet principles One to Six, but giving yourself full freedom of choice.

The question 'do I really want it?' is a really powerful one, especially for someone who's been living their life according to ingrained habits for years and years. That was me, when I began writing the original book.

I was married when I started writing it, and it transversed one of the most traumatic periods in my life as I ended up getting divorced in between finishing the original book and it going to press. There then followed a period of transition – major transition – which I go into further detail about here.

We all have a story – and this chapter covers the era of my life where I coped with:

- becoming a single mum
- getting used to being divorced
- starting up a whole business empire and seeing it crumble again
- being made redundant four times in two years (serve me right for working in the Finance industry. An ex-boyfriend ran a – yes you've guessed it – sub-prime mortgage company! Eeek! I'm coming out in hives just thinking about it…)
- … and about him. It wasn't a good period in my life, and I went through treatment for depression. And out the other side again.
- through it all, my kids were relying on me – solely me – to get them through their teenage years and university. Which I did. Alone. How brilliant.
- I had a couple of other boyfriends – including a 'tragically funny one night stand.' It was so funny, in fact, that it made it into one of my romance novels, as a never-to-be-repeated

experience for the heroine, Sadie. Another relationship started out with the guy declaring loudly he was a single man, yet he still pursued me, so 'Debbie the rescuer' clicked into 'fix him' mode (he was the one with the issues with cheese and cats. And money. And authority. And staying positive and hopeful.) Unfixable. *Eurgh.*

Needless to say I have totally learned from these experiences and view myself now as a wiser individual. And still ever hopeful of finding the right man to settle down with. 'One day...' you know the rest, regulars... '*When I'm a grown up*!'

Oh yes, I had my fair share of 'what was I thinking' eras. And it took its toll on my well-being. Here in this exclusive, I go into more detail about the whys and wherefores of what happened in the interim period - between the end of the last Till the Fat Lady Slims book (2002) and when my current crusade began, to get fit and slim again.

You'll also find in this book a short outline of my own ideal routine to get in shape – for those who really want to be guided – I've called it the 'DF Plan' diet! Hehe! Read on....

What Happened Next? 2000 - 2002

It was a funny time in my life, this one. I remember talking to a friend, Ali, about what she called my 'metamorphosis.' All the while I was writing the original 2002 TTFLS book (you'll read it in Part Three) I was actually going through a painful marriage break up.

I ended up finding out that after fourteen years, the husband and I had different ideas of what it took to make a marriage work. A year after we split up, I discovered he'd been playing around - for most of our marriage. Seriously.

The one thing it did do, was to give me the peace of mind that through it all, when I used to have suspicions, they were actually correct. So I knew I could trust my instincts after all.

At that time I was learning a lot about myself. I thoroughly recommend a lot of resources if you need to do the same – self-help books and audio books – from Wayne Dyer to Tony Robbins, Deepak Chopra to business books like Steven Covey and Kenneth Blanchard. The 'Seven Secrets of Successful People' was one of my faves, as '*seek first to understand then be understood*' became one of my mantras. As did Wayne Dyer's '*give up your need to be right*,' and '*be independent of the good and bad opinion of others*.' His way of dealing with people who disagree vehemently with your choices, changed my life at that point – when they told me they didn't like what I'd bought myself, or what I was doing with my life, I'd just say '*you'll get over it*'. And as I say in Part Three, dealing with those people differently makes such a difference to being able to carry on with your job of changing the habits of a lifetime.

'Cos the 'tribe' don't like it when a member steps outside the box.

Don't be scared to counter their objections. When you start saying 'actually I don't feel like it,' or 'not now, but I'd love to save one for later,' it will irk some people. But they'll get used to it…

Those around me took the mick initially. Specially people who poo-poo'ed most things – you know, the cynical ones. Or the ones who know it all, but never practise what they preach. But they soon changed their tune when they saw how my body was slimming down more than ever before. Finally a 'diet' that worked. Only it's not a diet. It's about as opposite from a controlled diet as you can get!

I realised there was no point trying to change the ones who were not ready. But eventually those very people would be coming to me asking how I'd done it, especially when I lost weight over Xmas one year.

The problem was, that was my last married Xmas.

I guess I found I could live my life without obeying his rules, after all. And of course he didn't accept that very easily. Previously I'd cave in to a situation, he'd get his way and I'd just go smother my emotion with food. Gradually it became the norm that I would stand up for myself instead, and battle to fix what was at the heart of the problem – the problem that previously caused my emotional eating.

Initially my independence was admired by him, and he was seemingly proud of what I was doing to change my shape – after all, he'd always kept himself trim and fit so it was something he admired. But then came the differences of opinion about the kids and their meal times. I began getting them to sit down at the table with me, rather than in front of the telly. I'd say 'ok' if they told me they'd had enough, whereas his reaction was stuck in his childhood – 'finish what's on your plate.' 'No,' I'd say, 'if they've had enough it's ok to leave it.' And at the same time, he'd started staying out at 'work' longer and longer, until our marriage reached breaking point once I moved up to Peterborough for a new job.

Yes, I left QVC. BUT in this brave new world of being completely independent again, I was ruling my own life, with no one else to worry about for half the week (the other half I was back down in the family home again, as that was the arrangement once we'd split up.)

I'd go to Frankie and Benny's on the estate near where the new studios were based, for lunch with some of the team, and obey the Slim Person's rules. Consequently I'd end up bringing home half the chicken, salad and chips to eat later. People soon got used to me.

I got used to me.

And I liked me.

I carried on losing the weight, and ended up being more slim and toned pushing forty, than I was in most of my thirties. In fact, at 36 I'd been my heaviest ever, and desperately unhappy. I knew I was an emotional eater – the 'binge' I describe in a later part of this book really happened. Some of you may not believe it – looking back now, I hardly believe it! How much food I ate at one sitting was scary. But it was happening – and all behind closed doors. So having left that person behind, I was damned if I was going to give her up easily.

Whilst up in Peterborough I went on a life-changing series of seminars and workshops by Tony Robbins. His stuff is still pretty mind-blowing, if you like that sort of thing. Yes, it's all a bit happy-clappy, but I was embracing it all back then – in truth it was exactly what I needed.

I went to Hawaii, on 'Life Mastery' and to Miami on 'Date with Destiny' and both these week-long workshops helped me grasp a much better understanding of how I tick.

So another thing I can take out of that era is that, if you want to change the habits of a lifetime, it won't be overnight. But with the right techniques, new habits can be formed. And a supportive environment is vital to enable you to continue the journey and not slip back to old ways.

In fact, it took me another few years, until a major upset in my life, for any slipping to occur.

Bad Business – 2002 - 2009

After a couple of years of being single, I'd pretty much got a grip on my new single life. At the end of the day, when the doors closed and the lights went off, I was as guilty as the next person of sitting listening to sad songs and hosting my own private pity-party.

I remember when Bridget Jones' Diary the movie came out, I saw it with a friend who declared 'that's you!' over and over again through the film. I had to laugh at the bit where poor thirty-something singleton Bridget feels sorry for herself, singing 'All by Myself.' My Whitney Houston CD got a pretty good bashing that year, I can tell you. But happily, shortly after that I was off to Hawaii. It was there that I discovered Penta Water.

Now if you read 'Hawaiian Affair,' my first steamy romance novel, you'll know that Sadie the heroine ends up running a special bottled water business. Well, it's not all fiction – the water bit, anyway. Sadie getting off with the millionaire investor was definitely all made up (sadly!), but much of the basis of how the water helped performance was inspired by the Penta Water story. I first encountered it on sale on a little table outside the main conference hall at Life Mastery in Hawaii.

Here I was, two years later in 2002, with an embryonic importing business, still dabbling in shopping telly (at another channel – I'd left Peterborough by now. In an ideal world I'd have stayed. But I discovered it wasn't one.)

The big leap to running my own business full time came with a canny connection from our then PR guru whom we'd hired to help publicise the previous shopping channel. He put me in touch with another of his clients, who was a venture capital investor. This guy was really interested in Penta after he found out it helped him avoid jet lag, and with his financing and encouragement, along with a wise financial advisor he put in place, called Philip, the fledgling 'Penta UK' was up and running. I was in and out of inconsequential relationships at that time, but at least I had my master plan – next year we'd all be millionaires! Not really, but at least with a sound business plan and some proper bank financing and all the usual things that go with retailing, I had a genuine prospect of making some serious money if we could tie down the exclusive contract for the UK. Hopes, dream, plans – you know the stuff. I had them all.

By early 2004 we had offices in Leatherhead, a small team of six or so, two business partners, about 500 retail outlets in the UK, (Waitrose came later), and enough finance for me to go full time. Our investor wanted proper marketing advice, so we employed a fabulous marketing company, who in turn put me in touch with a guy called Harry, CEO of a successful energy drinks brand. Harry became my mentor and I loved every second of being in charge of this embryonic gold mine. I was too busy to be lonely or resort to emotional eating.

Mark my sports director was bringing on sports teams and athletes, boat race crews and premier football teams, as well as top rugby clubs and celebrities. Even Tom Cruise was pictured with a Penta in his hand. The science was impressive, and by early 2005 we'd achieved an amazing feat – three UK university studies showing our water was definitely different.

Through it all, I'd maintained my Freedom Eating – and stayed roughly the same weight.

Yes there were stressful times, but after a short period of three months being vegan in 2000 for one of the Tony Robbins workshop challenges, I'd noticed how much better my body felt and after that I mainly stayed 'clean' eating – mostly veggie, and very few unhealthy foods, sweets etc, as I just didn't want them. Plus of course, lots of water! I was almost never ill.

Then things started to fall apart.

We were under big pressures to perform, under our new exclusive contract which we'd managed to obtain. Harry had helped impress the US parent company which manufactured Penta, and meeting our investor over in San Diego had sealed the deal – we were now the UK and Europe distributor. BUT – do you recall the Dasani bottled water debacle, around 2004? It made people wary of expensive water that needed an explanation. Our sales faltered. Then the parent company decided to tighten up their contract terms, as our sales weren't high enough. And without going into too much detail, as that's a book in itself, we floundered. By mid 2005, my business was wound up and with it, all the personal investment I'd made, meaning I too went bankrupt. There wasn't much option for an alternative and believe me I looked for another way. But with the blessing of our investor, we dissolved the company. He was a rock, and still is – we meet for coffee every so often even now.

But things looked bleak for me, financially. It was one of the most stressful times of my life, that's for sure.

At the same time, my boy was doing his A' levels, and getting ready to go to uni, and my girl was doing her GCSE's and moving to college. So whilst I was putting a brave face on it on the outside, I was hurting inside, big time, and my focus got a little off target.

There was a little light at the end of the tunnel, or so I thought, in the form of a 'rescuer' relationship. A new guy. A boyfriend – one who was the MD of a mortgage company, who worked in the same serviced offices as we did. We met to discuss our companies, swap advice etc, and it was clear he liked me. When he split from his wife of one year, he came straight to me, and I gladly accepted him, having previously refused to be party to any form of cheating. After all, I'd been on the receiving end of infidelity myself courtesy of my ex husband so I didn't want to inflict it on another woman.

Mr Mortgage and I forged ahead with a relationship, but I knew so early on it was doomed, I just didn't have the resources to cope with giving it up alongside everything else going wrong. He threw money at my problems, which frankly was a short term solution and a long term disaster. It didn't help my state of mind. I'd always been independent and it emasculated me. Which sounds strange, but considering I'd been the mum AND the dad for several years, and fiercely independent, it was making me feel useless to rely on someone else in that way. But I took that road as an easy option, which only made me feel worse. I didn't have much choice, not with Lauren still at home, watching her hapless mother conduct a love affair with a man eleven years my junior and who was blatantly obviously not right for me.

Mr Mortgage and I split up five times in the first year. And in just under two years, we had ever-more violent break ups, totalling twelve in all. It's too long a story for this book, and it's not entirely relevant to the theme. But I'm just setting the scene so you can understand how this major upheaval in my life led to my next phase. He and I parted twenty two months after we began, and about eighteen months later than we should have done.

By then I'd been working for him, and that ended too. My world kind of fell apart – all my own fault but it was made worse by being a victim of circumstance somewhat. And the word 'victim' and 'me' had never been in the same sentence. But fate dealt its hand, and if everything happens for a reason, I was damn sure I didn't know what it was at that time. I'd learned some major lessons, but was left being treated for depression.

Dealing with Depression

Yes, depression. Me.

No, I wouldn't have believed it either. But there it was, a little blister pack of Citalopram, small dose, taking me through six months I'd rather not ever repeat again in my life. They served a purpose, those little pills. Gave me some wicked dreams! But took about another two years to fully get out of my system. They definitely mucked up my brain chemistry. And put me in what I called 'citalopram neutral,' where nothing made me desperately sad any more, but nothing made me wonderfully happy either. Weird time.

When I'd begun my relationship with Mr Mortgage, amidst his talk of marriage and not wanting to have babies 'cos I already had them (what a load of tosh! He's married with two little ones now, LOL!), I found myself being bullied again, in the same way my ex husband had done years before. Only this time, with diminished confidence, I didn't have enough fight in me, and I began to get out of the habits of my precious Freedom Eating. Mr Mortgage would moan if I wasn't ready to eat when he'd made me dinner. He'd also want desserts and expect me to join in. He'd frequently make food his 'thing' and what with the tragic nature of our on/off relationship, my patterns of eating began to change. There's more to it than that – far more – but you get the idea.

After we ended, and my business had folded completely, I went off to work for another mortgage company, then another. Yes, they were sub-prime mortgage packagers. My new career was back in finance, where I'd begun, having taken a business degree at the London School of Economics when I was younger, to become a chartered accountant. So it wasn't a massive mismatch. Ironically I thoroughly enjoyed it.

At the time it was my lifeline – safe. A routine-based daily grind which gave me regular as clockwork hours and roles – was just what I needed at that time. Heck, I even found the highlight of my day was making my cup of tea with sugar in (lots) which I frequently made myself and drank throughout my working day. I managed a team of more than a dozen mortgage processors and learning the ins and outs of obtaining mortgages for people with less than perfect credit profiles. People like me.

I wasn't myself at all during that period. I recall one weekend when the kids were busy and I was at a loss for what to do with myself. I ended up deciding that the thing that would give me more pleasure than anything else was to go back in to work, armed with my manager's set of keys, and newly purchased bleach and cloths, and completely clean the grimy communal kitchen. Yes really. That was probably quite a low point in my life I must say. Coupled with that, I was slowly getting used to the typical office way of life. My lovely ladies would bring in home-made cakes. The wonderful mortgage lenders whom we worked with would send in tins of sweets every time a big deal came off. And it was always someone's birthday or event.

Gradually the weight crept back on.

I didn't notice it at first, but it hit home one time when I had a tragically funny one night stand. I won't go into great detail here, but as I've already mentioned it led to a particularly tragic love scene for one of my heroines in one of my novels. Although I held back on some of the detail. That's definitely for another book!

But I was quite large again by the time I managed to work my way back to QVC. That had happened via deciding to retrain for a different career, by obtaining Prince 2 professional operations management qualifications, which led to a job as a manager at another shopping channel and they had me back on air by Xmas. It was like shopping telly saying 'you can't escape meeeee!' No surprise then, that finally, after nine years away, I managed to visualize hard enough that the powers that be at QVC decided it was time for me to return.

But I'd just had time off for a mini op on my waterworks, two weeks of sitting still recovering, followed soon after by my first ever writing workshop – in Tuscany, eating amazing food but too much of it – pasta and desserts, and late night snacks as we all learned about 'show not tell' and sub-plots and head hopping. I came back pretty big. Again. I'd never resumed binge-eating, that was one blessing.

Back at QVC, Back to Me – 2009 - 2014

I knew I had to do something, but what? By now I was back at QVC. It was lovely doing Thornton's chocolate hours, or eating delicious yogurts for a whole hour, but I'd got too far removed from Principle 6. And there lay the problem. I realised it was probably sugar. I had got pretty unfit too. So I had to do something that worked...

A weight loss programme called Diet Chef helped and I lost a stone, and if you do what it says, it works. But for me, as you've probably guessed, I have trouble with the 'doing what it says' bit. So I put it gradually back on again. Sure, those systems work – they work for many who can follow a plan – and if you can too, that's great. (Or, if you quite like following a plan but need extra help, or you'd like it to feel easier, well that's where the 'When' Diet comes in – just do both concurrently.)

But I still personally can't diet. As I keep saying, if someone tells me 'you can't,' it's like a red rag to a bull – because then I want to – whatever 'it' is, even if I didn't want to beforehand.

By Summer 2011 my daughter had finished uni and announced she was staying in Bath and wouldn't be moving back home any more. I'd got into the habit of feeding the loneliness with tea and biscuits. And looking back it was easy to see over the years why it had slipped.

For me, the crunch came soon after. I was getting nearer 50 and finding it hard to breathe deeply, almost all of the time. I was climbing over stiles whilst dog walking, or doing certain yoga positions, and finding I couldn't breathe in at all, whilst bending my knees up to my chest. Something was wrong inside my body and I didn't like it. Looking back now, I'm sure I had the start of a condition called Fatty Liver. Google it, it's not nice. I'd got into the habit over the years of relying too much on sugar in my coffee, and packets of biscuits whilst alone late at night after working all day at my job. (Lots of different jobs – I really must write that full autobiography one day!)

A newspaper ad talked about a workshop in April 2012 in Scotland run by Marlene Watson Tara (.com) where you learned how to cook yourself the best nutrition possible. So I went. And found a much healthier way of eating... of living... of being. After a couple of years spent expanding my knowledge about plant based, wholefood diets, macrobiotics and 'doctor nutrition,' plus finding out about the foods my body didn't like. Since then I've given up almost all dairy, most meat and much wheat, plus I've added essential elements from a macrobiotic influence. (see later – the 'DF Plan.') All in all, I turned a corner as far as being able to decline 'bad' foods. I was also getting better at turning down 'bad' men.

I finished that awful relationship with the cheese-eating, cat allergy man, (a whole 'nother source of despondency!) and went back to full Freedom Eating. Only this time, armed with the extra info and resources I've listed below in Part Two – a whole stack of research to help expand our understanding of the body and how it works, so we can interpret the signals correctly and do Principle 6 right.

Now, Winter 2014 - What do I do?

I've lost weight again, and am continuing to lose, and at the same time I'm toning up with the help of some wicked QVC fitness devices and yoga and dog walks. Because there's actually a seventh principle – and that is to do in life what you feel your body – and you – really need. From meditation to walking to cutting loose from relationships that no longer serve you. If we listen to that tiny voice inside us giving us advice, often it's right. I do hope whichever element of this system you choose, it really helps you get 'Back to You' – the 'you' you were born to be, before society, a lifetime of dieting – and fructose – intervened.

Enjoy the rest of this updated book, Till the Fat Lady Slims 2.0 – The 'When' Diet. It was specially written just for you, the new generation of Freedom Eaters! And everlasting thanks to Sean and Vicky the originators for the legacy they left me that's now transforming so many new lives, all over again .

EXTRA MATERIAL – can be found on my website

www.debbieflint.co.uk/TTFLS

BONUS EXCLUSIVE MATERIAL for readers of this book –

www.debbieflint.co.uk/BONUS

enter password code TTFLSQVC2015 where prompted

Let me know your progress – debbie@debbieflint.com

27th July – sister Linda Bignell – ex slimming club leader, on TTFLS

"When my sis gave me her book in 2002 I read it and felt liberated! Always a member of Weight Watchers I would count and weigh and often override my body in judging the obvious! .... So although I still weigh once a week! (Just can't let go!!!) I now listen to myself! What does my body WANT to eat? Stopping when I'm satisfied ...... Being more active..... Smaller plates and portions!......I'm 50 now and I'm not trapped in diet prison anymore! I take the best of freedom eating skills and combine it with healthy choices."

On combining Freedom Eating with Christmas and Vacations

"For maintenance it's amazing. The biggest thing that it did for me, was that it changed what I did at Xmas and on holidays. Rather than thinking 'it's Xmas I can overeat,' I was thinking 'what do I really want, and if I want it I can have it?' The same as on my holiday. Having it when I wanted it meant it was making me stop far, far earlier and I wasn't overeating. The usual chocolates tasted waxy and weren't hitting the spot. I remember the first Xmas I did it, I didn't put on so much weight as usual.

I do the same thing when I go on holiday – there's nothing that's out of bounds. I'm not thinking 'Oh God, I'm on holiday, it's all inclusive, I've got to stuff my face!' I'm having it when I want it. And not obsessing about it. I often want vegetables, even at breakfast time, so the buffets were heaven and I came back for the first time without having gained a pound.

Therefore it could be a big part of what people do when they've lost the weight they want to lose. That's me now. For me, it's now not a 'diet,' I call it my plan. When I ran slimming classes, nine times out of ten, the very overweight people were eating to compensate for something that was missing in their lives. For them, learning the WHEN Plan will be a revelation. They should also not be scared of hunger – it's part of normal life as long as it's used in the right way. It's certainly changing lives."

Go to www.debbieflint.com/TTFLS for a podcast of our whole chat.

PART TWO – Further Resources & the 'DF Plan!'

a. Sugar Prison

My sister arrived at my house one day. Her son Ricky was training to be an osteopath and had told her about a video doing the rounds. So I reluctantly watched it. And it changed my life.

Fructose – it's a chronic poison. Or so says a particularly adamant university professor in a ninety minute recording of a Uni lecture that became a 'sensation' between 2004 and 2010. I'd been back at QVC a year, and I watched *'Sugar the Bitter Truth'* the YouTube video by Professor Robert Lustig in October 2010. After the fourth time (I kept getting my loved ones to watch it with me so I saw it over and over till it sank in), I gave up sugar completely. That Christmas, Andrew the guest from Gatineau, the beauty brand, gave each presenter five small Champagne Truffles in a pack. I'd had a particularly tough shift on a charity day and having been sugar-free for about a month I decided I'd 'trial' eating one. Then another. And another and another and another. That felt OK, I thought. For a short while. Then after a sugar high, I had the most horrendous crash and unbelievable sickness and headaches – a sugar hangover - for three days afterwards. I'm not kidding.

A year or so later, during the tail end of a relationship going bad, when sugar started to creep back in again to my diet, I found myself giving in to temptation and without realising it, it grasped me. I had a Christmas of being quite big – and quite ill. Lots of migraines and lots of not being able to breathe very well. I found that at work (on air at QVC) on a kitchen show if I ate lots of very sweet popcorn or one of Simon Brown's bowls of upside down sponge puddings one day, that I swiftly got dragged back in like a quagmire the next. My body was being taken over like a demon, and began desiring more sugary stuff.

So I went on a healthy eating workshop in Scotland and the information I learned completely focussed me on how to more effectively do Principle Six – be an observer not a judge – and pay attention to how food can both cause as well as cure illness.

I actually learned a really interesting subject, all about how macrobiotic eating could solve so many issues. Within a week I was breathing more clearly having given up dairy and excess added sugar, meat and simple carbs. OMG did I feel healthy after! Within a month my skin began to glow, and after having had progressively fewer and farther apart periods (close your ears guys) I then had three periods exactly 28 days apart. Unheard of for me, yet it was happening - something good was clearly going on in my body.

Talk about Doctor Nutrition! Or Food Medicine. Whatever it was, my hormones were balancing, my biome was regenerating and I had no more aching hands and joints in the morning.

It revolutionised my beliefs about what is possible in an ageing body. Any ageing body. We can all make the best of what we've got. Some things cannot be cured, but some things can – if you only know what to do. If you've ever found a product that changed your life, think about how you felt beforehand, when you didn't know about it. If someone had told you the change would happen would you have scoffed at them? But now you know better, right? Well, maybe, just maybe, there are some things that you're eating which are causing the issues you have. And maybe just maybe there are some things you could start eating which could help prevent the issues you have.

For me, now, I only get aching joints if I eat 'crap' food – swollen knuckles in the mornings – symptoms of 'arthritis? Well dad had it, God rest him, so no doubt I would have it too. That is if I didn't eat what I eat, and take what I take (high EPA) and avoid what I avoid. Talking of which – see below about the information regarding omega 3 fish oils and their many benefits to the body.

There are other videos to watch which will help you wise up about sugar on YouTube including (at time of writing) these:

- 'Toxic sugar'
- 'Is sugar toxic, a sixty minutes report' and
- 'Sugar the bitter truth' with Prof Robert Lustig. The granddaddy of them all. If you're having real genuine problems banishing your sugar cravings – especially if you're an intelligent person and you love finding out information – find out about addictive fructose and its effect on the body.

It's worth a try – search the titles and watch them several times.

After all, you can't say it doesn't work for you unless you give it a go, can you? And once your body is free of the sugar addiction, you'll find many of the principles of Freedom Eating so much easier to follow.

a. A Word about Fat v Sugar

Here is some other info about diet myths you may still believe to be true – new information has come out about low fat diets and it pays to be wise.

Professor Robert Lustig is the guru of fructose-avoidance-theory and in his 2013 book, *Fat Chance: the Bitter Truth About Sugar,* and on his YouTube video mentioned above, he also explains in layman's terms how the health advisors in the USA got it tragically wrong in 1982 when the FDA began the 'low fat' campaign; it should have been 'low fat AND low sugar.'

Since then, the epidemic of metabolic syndrome has happened – showing this advice had the opposite effect of what the FDA intended. Why? Because manufacturers taking out the fat were replacing it with sugar. Just because it's lower fat, DOES NOT mean it's healthier. Check the labels. Anything over 5% sugar content should be severely restricted.

That's not to say 'never have it', IF saying that to yourself means you binge on it. See Principles 1-6 in The 'When' Diet! But if you're being sensible and using knowledge to benefit your quest for better health and a slimmer body, it's worth investigating this research. If you're like me, it helps me not WANT these high sugar foods. And a funny thing happens – when sugar is out of my system for a while, the higher sugar foods actually DON'T taste so good any more. My body doesn't want them – and neither does my brain. Especially since I found out how officialdom got it so wrong.

Google it. Everything that's happened since 1982 could have been totally avoided. It still can, if you get high fructose out of your diet. For instance, Rob Lustig says fruit juices are a no-no – eat the whole fruit, since the fibre it contains is also the antidote. And don't eat too much fruit in any case. Fruits with high sugar and low fibre are going to make you put on weight and any diet which says fruit is unlimited, but doesn't differentiate between different types, is out of date.

The only place fructose can be metabolised is in the liver. A third of all calories consumed from fructose are converted into fat. No matter what else you eat or what exercise you do, it'll happen. His 'Sugar the bitter truth' video shows exactly how, for the intelligent students amongst you (it's an hour and a half long and features much biochemistry). Or, just read his amazing book to see why it's so vital to make the changes to your diet now. If everyone did it, it would take society out of this destructive spiral of burgeoning health costs, he says. And any doctor who doesn't ask you about your nutrition when you go in for many common major illnesses, needs to also study Rob Lustig's work too. In fact, in summer 2014, it hit the news that key medical experts were calling for GPs to be more educated in nutrition. About time!

People like Professor Lustig and his peers are revolutionising public awareness about food and how it can harm, and how it can cure. The info is out there – go Google, people!

b. Omega 3 Fish Oils

Doctor Alexandra Richardson is another one. She's the Oxford professor who did those very first Durham school trials on omega 3, showing how children with certain attention issues can be helped with supplementation of extra EPA (an omega 3 from fish oil). This created the massive boom in omega 3 products.

Now I'm not going to say 'take loads of supplements, they're the best thing ever.' Ideally we'd all get everything we need from a balanced diet. BUT IF YOU DON'T, let me inform you about some of the information I've discovered. Much of which comes under the heading of 'Principle 6.'

Some of it changed my daughter's life as far as eczema was concerned. I'm not a doctor, and this is not doctor's advice, but as it's a semi-autobiographical weight loss book, I'm continuing with my own story and journey of discovery.

In the mid 2000s my small importing company (Penta Water – see previously) had migrated into a promotions company helping health food industry firms create marketing materials. One contract was for a fish oils brand. In the process I became friends with Dr Alex Richardson. She told me, as only learned scientists can, about the massive impact on the body of EPA (and to a lesser extent DHA,) both a type of omega 3 from fish oils. Her current findings have since increased – now she gives talks about the research showing how omega 3 (EPA/DHA) can help hair, nails, skin, eyes, the brain, focus, concentration, sleep, depression, ADHD, the immune system, cholesterol, blood pressure, inflammation of all kinds, the heart, pregnant women (DHA), children under 5 (DHA) etc, etc.

Erm, that's kind of... almost everything, right?

So - I could eat lots of oily fish from a non-pcb, non-dioxin, non-mercury source (hard but not impossible) or I could take high quality fish oils, which I now do. (Which ones? I sometimes mention what supplements I take on my website blog – Back to You page.)

More importantly, so does Lauren my daughter, who suffered from awful debilitating eczema during much of her childhood. She takes it in high doses, (2000mg) every day. This, along with avoiding SLS (sodium laureth or lauryl sulphates) in shower gels, helps her eczema stay under control, having tried EVERTHING in her youth to no avail. When she was about 16, suddenly we had the solution to her eternally scratchy, itchy, red, sore arms, legs, and bottom-cheeks, and a life of being covered with thick creams each night came to an end. She literally gained her confidence back and blossomed.

I tell you – if only I'd known all that when she was 4! Then I began more than a decade of trying every known cream and tablet and Chinese herb under the sun. I'm OK with SLS but she's not. And when she avoids that, and takes her high EPA each day, she's mostly on the straight and narrow, on the whole. This is her experience, it won't be the same for everybody. Info can affect your choices. Just be wise.

Dr Alex Richardson talks about people who have brought down both their blood pressure and high cholesterol with enough EPA, and the studies Alex showed me examined depression victims and violent prisoners as well as disruptive school children, all of whom were massively affected by taking enough high dose EPA. Arthritis as well, can be hugely helped by it, she said.

So check with your expert but then go Google. And if the expert says 'I don't know of any proof' then they simply may not know of it. There are many not paying attention to nutrition news, and just handing out old advice – and tablets – willy-nilly for all sorts of issues. Marlene Watson Tara's amazing blogs talk about diabetes and some very serious illnesses, and the effect of pure plant-based diets. Also, that according to the World Health Organisation, the vast majority of some of the world's top serious illnesses are nutrition based, or rather 'lack of nutrition' based.

It really is a whole new world out there – hence this update to the original 'Till the Fat Lady Slims' book from 2002. The main principles still hold, and the semi-autobiographical bit (until 2002) remains. If you don't know what happened to me when I first began Freedom Eating, read part 3 – TTFLS original. Maybe your story will be the same as mine.

What do I do? The 'DF Plan'

On Facebook many have requested a list of what I do, and have done, exactly, precisely, and entirely, in order that they may follow it too.

The idea is you eventually find what works for you, so if you're able to promise yourself and me that this is only an initial guide, here it is – the 'Debbie Flint Plan,' or the 'DF Plan!'

Daily Diet

- tons of fresh veg, salad, a miso soup each day, a stir fry with greens most days (recipe at end of this segment,) sweet vegetable tea (see marlenewatsontara.com for recipe,) to help combat sugar cravings, seaweed strips for snacks (from asian section in big supermarkets,) some nuts each day but not too many (don't want to overdo it with the omega 6 as it reduces the good ratio of 6:3 in the body) lots of fresh water (not tap) and my favourite supplements:

- I avoid dairy, most meat and much wheat. I eat fish and eggs.

- I take high dose EPA fish oils (1500mg a day of actual EPA) plus Vitamin C, CoQ10 and a good multi-vitamin. But also I've been impressed with Imedeen supplements - between January and April my skin density went from 47 to 53, a ten per cent improvement!

- if needed, a green superfood drink (eg Barleans Greens – a powder you take in water. Contains roots and shoots and berries and leaves and grasses etc. Or similar – tons available online.) Once a day or as often as needed – more if under the weather

- I practise meditation, I walk my dogs daily and every night before bed I do a three minute yoga stretch – a version of sun salutations.

- I have stepped up my bodyblade use, doing, at minimum, the ex No.6 hip and thigh for one full minute a day, giving the last 15 seconds all I can – that's what really works. Plus one minute leg master. I love the rebounders and if you can get one, the Pilates Reformer is top notch

- I only have me to worry about most of the time, and my three Labradors. I'm lucky, I know, hard work is done! But worth mentioning.

Suggested Induction - The 'DF Plan

Week One – Introduce the 'When' Diet principles gradually.

- begin by giving your food your full attention
- try stopping at satisfied not full, as often as you can
- definitely don't feel guilty if you have 'bad' foods – think, 'does my body really want them? If so, have them but stop at satisfied.

Week Two –

- pay attention to being properly hungry – only eat at 6
- continue to stop at satisfied, and aim to get it right
- experiment with what effect different foods have on you

Week Three –

- now focus on food choices. Hold out for the ones which really sing to you.
- Ensure you're waiting till 6 on hunger scale still before eating
- Ensure you're stopping at satisfied – carry a container round with you to put leftovers in for later when hungry enough again

Week Four –

- Put it all into practise, every day, rigorously
- Resist the influence of others, get used to the new habit of paying attention to your body's needs.
- If you're brave enough, stop weighing yourself
- Join Till the Fat Lady Slims TTFLS Facebook group and report your progress! Leave a review for book on Amazon or Goodreads – thank you!

Research and Further Reading 2014

Go to my website www.debbieflint.com to the Back to You tab, where you'll see a weekly well-being blog and an archive that's an armoury of info including so many helpful studies. Eg, showing how we can shed cravings

http://drhyman.com/blog/2012/03/01/how-to-rewire-your-brain-to-end-food-cravings/

http://www.mydaily.co.uk/2014/09/03/how-to-train-your-brain-to-love-low-calorie-foods/?ncid=wsc-uk-mydaily-headline

Books

'What are you Hungry For' – Deepak Chopra – @deepakchopra - fab exploration of the causes of emotional eating

'Escape the Diet Trap' – Dr John Briffa – @drbriffa - more of what I've touched upon here, but from a doctor's point of view, and full of fantastic links to studies, research and science. Can you tell I'm a science geek!?

'They are What You Feed Them' – Dr Alexandra Richardson – also https://www.facebook.com/**FABResearch** If anyone knows what your kids should be eating, she does.

'Macrobiotics for All Seasons' – Marlene Watson Tara – @marlenewt - macrobiotics queen explains why we need to eat like our ancestors. Her website, including a fabulous sweet vegetable tea to help combat sugar cravings, is www.marlenewatsontara.com

'Fat Chance – the Bitter Truth About Sugar' - Professor Robert Lustig – @robertlustigMD (it's all about the sugar, people!')

So do your research – go Google.

PART THREE –

Till the Fat Lady Slims

(TTFLS 2002 Original version)

abridged

By Debbie Flint

First published 2002

TILL THE FAT LADY SLIMS (2002) - abridged

This was me in 1999...

There's this woman who is the same as countless others of the same age. Always said she'd be different. Always knew she'd achieve something special in her life; whether a superstar career girl, mother, friend, lover or naturally, a brilliant combination of all those. And she will be it - she has no doubt - one day. But first she just has to lose some weight. She's been saying it for some time now. In fact, trying to get a grip on the whole personal lifestyle thing. If she can - no - when she can do this, everything will be perfect. Everything will fall into place. Everything will start to happen.

Others like her have been saying it for years. And no one's ever contradicted her or made her think anything's amiss with her plan. Partly because she doesn't really discuss it all openly, just the dieting bit, and for many of them, that's accepted logic anyway: everyone diets don't they? In fact, everywhere she looks there's only reinforcement for her philosophy - from her friends and family, from all the knowledge at her fingertips, from the media, from those perfect examples of 'before and after' that magazine and newspapers frequently publish. They all say the same thing - the weight will go when she stops eating so much of the wrong thing - whatever 'wrong thing' is in vogue right now. When she cuts back on calories, or fat grams, carbohydrates or points, units or whatever - carefully counting and controlling - each new type of diet comes and goes, but there's always the next one. Yes, when she finds a diet plan that works, when she's 'good' and 'good' permanently - that's when it will all fall off and life can really begin again.

And she knows what it feels like to be 'good' – on the rare occasion she can call herself that, she's counting things, depriving and controlling - and maybe exercising consistently. That's good. Oh, and not smoking, or drinking too much, or arguing, or crying too often, or neglecting her friends/family/career - if she's really honest, that's really being 'good.' But it has to start with the right diet. And she knows that one day, in fact, one day soon, she'll be good all the time. After this next bad phase, in fact, right after it. NEXT TIME everything will work out. Isn't it always the way? So she'll just get this next bad phase out of the way, and happy days will be just around the corner, because only when she's good all the time is she allowed to be happy. But staying good all the time is oh, so hard. Oh she's convinced herself that next time it'll last, she'll get it right, but in truth, she's never stayed good all the time.

She knows it's really her fault, she knows the rules and she's the one who's broken them, so *she's* the one to blame - not *the rules*. Everyone knows *the rules*, and what happens when you break them. You're 'bad'. And you just need to be good - all the time - and then everything will fall into place. Everything will start to happen the way she knows it could. If she was good. All the time. But right now, as you read this, she's just in one of her bad phases. It'll pass.

Of course there are other options - the get slim quick products and ideas and fads. If she did those successfully, followed yet another set of rules then those options would bring her happiness sooner. Cabbage soup every day; eat only protein, take these tablets, use that lotion, this machine - all the time. Yes, she could use those solutions, follow them thoroughly and be good at them, too - *all the time*. But she doesn't. So the half-finished tubs of pills and potions are still in the cabinet. The half-read books are still by the bed. The machine's back in its box (or loaned to a friend - Good Samaritan, right?) The exercise routine lasted a little while, then she found she ran out of time each day. The ‘choose this not that', 'eat now not then' diet was too boring/difficult/ tasteless/ expensive/ anti-social, so it, too, went by the wayside. Eventually, in the scheme of things, she's become a font of all knowledge – she knows the rules, but she *doesn’t do them.* Why not? Well, *no way* was it the diet's/ tablet's/ potion's/machine's, regime’s or book's fault. Of course not, ‘cos they all worked – for a while. So they must work - it's just they did not work for her. Because *she's to blame*. Of course! Because she didn't do it right - she couldn't be good - *all the time.*

Well, what if there was a different kind of "good all the time", and it was easy? And it meant that over time, you would lose the weight, and therefore get the life you're meant to have, and you could achieve the ultimate goal - to be happy every day.

It's called Freedom Eating.

It’s not a fancy technique or a passing phase - it's how slim people live and it's just going back to basics. What your body's been trying to tell you for all those years, through all those rules your brain introduced, through all the socialisation concerning food deprivation and control you've learned along the way. This is how you start listening to your body all over again. It's how to reclaim your right to be happy. This is the way you should be naturally - the way some people are – the way slim people are. But not you. Not yet.

But *you can be*. And it all begins with reclaiming your natural birth-right to be slim. It's as natural as breathing. It's what your body was designed for. And the first step is Freedom Eating, and the extras I have added to it to create Food Freedom. If you read and re-read this book, and introduce it to your life, you can break free from Food Prison forever, and become that person you've kept on hold for years.

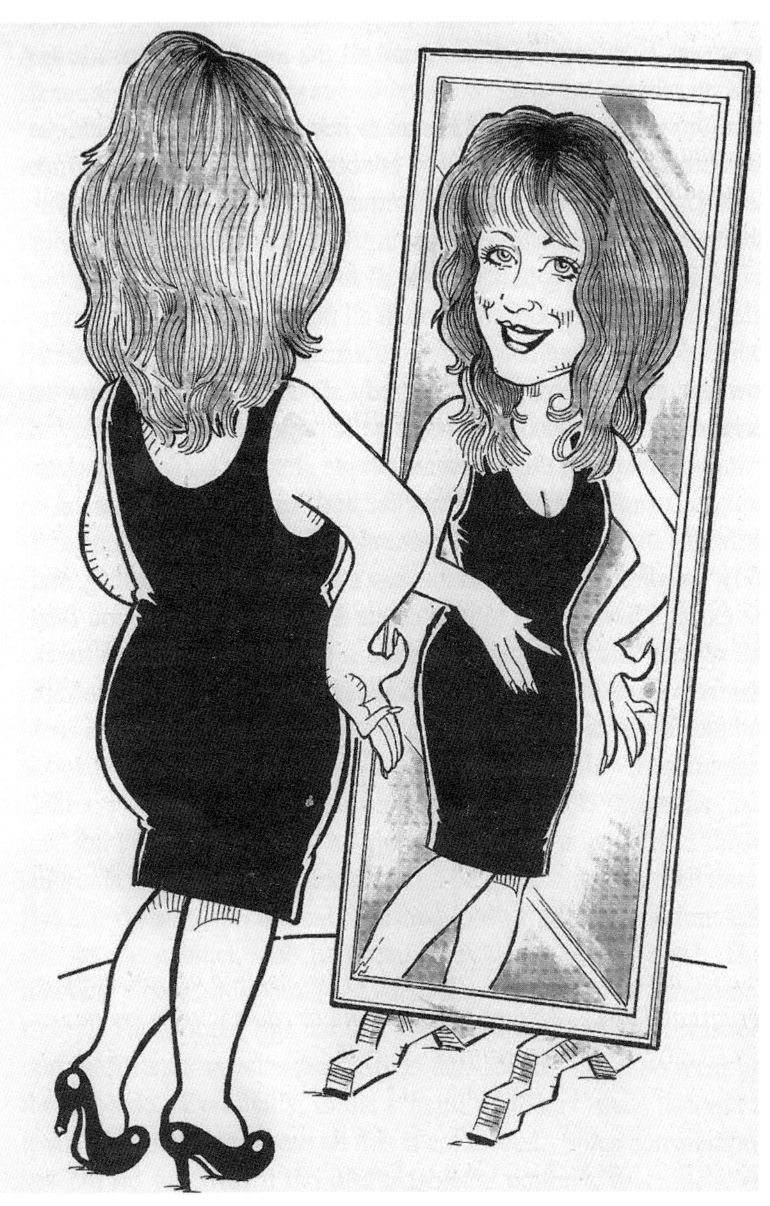

What do YOU see...?

Where it all Began c.1999

"When we first met Debbie, she was the top performing host at QVC, UK, and we were going on to present our product, Freedom Eating, a non-diet weight loss program. Debbie blew into the Green Room, full of enthusiasm. She had tried Freedom Eating since the previous time we had been on QVC and was steadily and easily losing weight! In fact, Debbie would do each show with us with a carefully balanced tower of lard bricks stationed next to her chair. She would command the cameras to zoom into the pile of lard bricks. "Each brick represents one pound of fat that I've lost on Freedom Eating," totalling, at that time 22 pounds. Today, of course it's much more weight than that. Debbie's success with Freedom Eating inspired many of her loyal QVC followers to try it. Freedom Eating. Within a couple of weeks of our QVC shows with Debbie hosting us for the first time, we were swamped with letters from thrilled women whose lives were being changed by Freedom Eating. Debbie's belief in - and experience with - the Freedom Eating approach has single-handedly influenced thousands and thousands of women to follow in her footsteps in the UK. Finally, Debbie has decided to tell her own story. And what a story it is!

One we all can relate to! You too will be inspired as you share in her ups and downs on the way to getting freedom with food and her ideal body. Freedom Eating began in the United States in 1986 when we tried to discover the secrets of becoming "naturally slim." To do this, we observed how naturally slim people ate and then copied their behaviours. As a result, we each lost over three stone, and have kept it off for fifteen years, without dieting at all.

In 1997, we published the book, The Seven Secrets of Slim People, and in 1999 created the Freedom Eating program which became available on videos and audio cassettes, as well as in the book. Through frequent media coverage on TV, radio and in magazine articles, the Freedom Eating message began to catch on. For the last three years, Freedom Eating has been widely marketed on the shopping channels in the US and UK, and many thousands of people's lives have been changed forever.

And now, we thank you Debbie for sharing your powerful story with the world."

Vikki Hansen and Shawn Goodman, authors of 7 Secrets of Slim People and creators of the original Freedom Eating system.

About The Author c.2001

Debbie Flint trained as an accountant, and took a business degree at the London School of Economics before entering the world of TV and Radio. Having started her broadcasting career at Piccadilly Radio in Manchester, from the same stable as Chris Evans, Steve Penk and Timmy Mallett, Debbie became the first female presenter in the Children's BBC Broom Cupboard. That was followed by the birth of her two children, stints on Open Air on BBC1, Living's 'Live at Three' and ten years with Children's SSVC TV Forces' Television. In 1998, Debbie returned to BBC1 to host her own game show Meet the Challenge. However, Debbie is probably best known from her work on UK Shopping Television - including QVC. There, in 1999, she came across the book and tape pack from Vikki Hansen and Shawn Goodman about the method of natural weight loss called **Freedom Eating**. Having used it herself to great effect, and due to viewers' requests, Vikki and Shawn asked her to write her own version, which was then picked up by Sahara Publications Limited.

The following is the original abridged version of the first Till the Fat Lady Slims book (2002.)

Enter the Fat Lady

Is this you?

January 2001

It's when you look at the photo and don't recognise yourself. When you see your inner self in the mirror because the external version is too alien to accept. When comfort eating is not just the solution, it's the beginning, the middle and the end of every day. That's when the fat lady has well and truly arrived. And you don't have to be outwardly 'fat' to have a fat lady take over your mind. How many of us hear someone we know saying, "I'm too fat, I need to lose at least ooh, five pounds," and watch in stunned disbelief as they grip at a mere half an inch or so of paltry pudge around their middle, knowing that we'd win this game hands down with our three or four rolls of at least an inch or two each.

We're fat. We know it. We just don't know what to do about it

Well for starters, how about looking into your past, at the behaviours society taught you, the rules and regulations you learned, the control and deprivation your mind lives its life by. All as a result of what we were told as we grew. There are people untouched by these habits. They are the slim people. The skinnies. The "I can eat anything I want" brigade, who make our already inadequate self-image even more resentful and controlling and scared. We haven't a clue how they can leave one mouthful of a chocolate bar, or the last bite of a burger, or the final pea on their plate. Or how they've been known to skip a meal. How they can say they don't want any dessert. Or how they can resist the temptation to share that oozing creamy birthday cake one day, yet tuck into a whole half a packet of biscuits the next. Without ever seeming to put on a pound. Well, guess what? I've studied these slim people. And I've found out how. I've looked at what they do to stay at their ideal weight, whilst eating normally. **It's called Food Freedom. And now you can do it too.**

The Seven Secrets of Slim People, and the associated tape programme, has helped thousands of people on both sides of the Atlantic to finally break free from food prison, to start living normal lives around food, and to gradually lose weight in the easy, enjoyable, favourite-food-filled process.

For me, it's meant turning the clock back ten years. Losing two and a half stone (35 pounds or so) naturally, and having my self-respect and dignity back. It's not a quick fix. It's not a temporary solution. It's not aided by tablets or injections or mad exercise regimes. It's not a guide to what to eat when, and how much it should measure. It's a practical, common sense step to permanent Food Freedom. And whether you adjust to it gradually, step by step, starting off alongside your diet, or go the whole hog immediately, this method can be used by everybody. Absolutely everybody.

It'll free you up to be the person you deserve to be and bring you the body you were meant to have naturally, had you never interfered with it, and affect those closest to you as they too emulate your behaviour. **Food Freedom means happier, slimmer kids too.**

So what do you say? Give it a go? All I ask is that you don't just read or listen once. The information you're about to read and hear about doesn't work unless you use it. Like anything, there are things that will rest easily with your lifestyle, and there may be things that don't work for you initially. Just do whatever feels right for you. Once you start really understanding what your body wants - with food at first - you'll end up in a better place than you ever thought possible, and so will your family. It's the first step to Freedom Living - and that's a real eye-opener, I can tell you. So if you've ever dreamed of that elusive, all-consuming freedom not to ever count another calorie, fat gram, carb unit or point not to ever have to step on the scales to decide whether you're going to have a good or a bad day, and not to ever have to follow the strangling, restricting, uncomfortable rules you've been led to believe are the only ones available to you concerning food, read on.

The secret food prisoner

There's this woman who is the same as countless others of the same age. Always said she'd be different. Always knew she'd achieve something special in her life; whether a superstar career girl, mother, friend, lover or naturally, a brilliant combination of all those. And she will be it - she has no doubt - one day. But first she just has to lose some weight. She's been saying it for some time now. In fact, trying to get a grip on the whole personal lifestyle thing. If she can - no - when she can do this, everything will be perfect. Everything will fall into place. Everything will start to happen.

Others like her have been saying it for years. And no one's ever contradicted her or made her think anything's amiss with her plan. Partly because she doesn't really discuss it all openly, just the dieting bit, and for many of them, that's accepted logic anyway: everyone diets don't they? In fact, everywhere she looks there's only reinforcement for her philosophy - from her friends and family, from all the knowledge at her fingertips, from the media, from those perfect examples of 'befores and afters' magazine and newspapers frequently publish. They all say the same thing - the weight will go when she stops eating so much of the wrong thing - whatever 'wrong thing' is in vogue right now. When she cuts back on calories, or fat grams, carbohydrates or points, units or whatever - carefully counting and controlling - each new type of diet comes and goes, but there's always the next one. Yes, when she finds a diet plan that works, when she's 'good' and 'good' permanently - that's when it will all fall off and life can really begin again.

Well, what if there was a different kind of "good all the time", and it was easy? And it meant that over time, you would lose the weight, and therefore get the life you're meant to have, and you could achieve the ultimate goal - to be happy every day.

It's called Freedom Eating.

It's not a fancy technique or a passing phase - it's how slim people live and it's just going back to basics. What your body's been trying to tell you for all those years, through all those rules your brain introduced, through all the social conditioning - food deprivation and control - you've learned since you were young. Right here is how you start listening to your body all over again. It's how to reclaim your right to be happy - the way you should be naturally - the way some people are – the way slim people are. Not you - not yet.

But *you can be*. And it all begins with reclaiming your natural birthright to be slim. It's as natural as breathing. It's what your body was designed for. And the first step is Freedom Eating, and the extras I have added to it to create Food Freedom. If you read and re-read this book, and introduce it to your life, you can break free from Food Prison forever, and become that person you've kept on hold for years.

Chapter One – In the World of the Fat

How long have you lived like this? Were you as bad as me...?

Surely someone who gets up in the middle of the night to rake the bin for leftovers can't be normal...

It was 1984. I was 22. Guests had come and gone and now the urges began. The *Spag Bol* wasn't so tempting, but skinny Jackie's barely touched jacket potato - still squashy with melted butter - was calling my name, loud. So as usual I replied, fished it out of the bin, and had a couple of minutes of heaven, devouring it alone in the dark. No one would know, no one would see, so it would all be ok, right? Except that it was *never* ok, and it was never enough. Afterwards, there was always that empty hole inside still waiting to be filled - a hole that not even the congealed, cold, spaghetti bolognaise could touch. But I had to find out, just in case. After all, this time was the Very Last Time wasn't it? The diet starts again tomorrow, and this time I'll stick to it. *Sound familiar?*

Yup, at time of writing that was fifteen years ago. And for all that time, *and* for most of the ten before that, I considered myself to have a weight problem. But I didn't, not at the start anyway. I was just a normal kid with a few podgy bits. But no one convinced me that I didn't need to think I had this weight problem and I watched adults around me and their dieting behaviour. And I obeyed the commands to finish the plate and treat sugary treats as reward and comfort. So it became a food problem. Which became a big problem once I got into my own house, living all on my own.

I could do what I wanted, when I wanted, with whom I wanted, and eat all the leftovers the morning after. And all the while I'd be going on every diet under the sun to try to lose the weight. The F-plan diet, the cabbage diet, the fasting diet, the hi-carb diet, the low-carb diet, the high protein diet, the detox diet, the Beverly Hills diet, and the seafood diet. Yes, some nights even Terry the Jolly Lodger was in danger if he sat still too long. Each one worked at the start, and then didn't. With every new fad, or 'technique', my search for that instant solution was running out of options and none of them worked permanently. In fact, the only thing I achieved was a weight loss yo-yo that damaged my self-esteem, annihilated my self-image, and set in motion a downward spiral of abstaining and bingeing punctuated by the 'lose a few, gain a few more' pattern we all know so well, plus a long-running series of dreams about missing out on food. How was I to know it would take another fifteen years before I came across a solution so powerful, it has literally transformed people's lives?

Nowadays, I look back on those times with mixed emotions. Independence brings with it a greater cost than many a trainee grown-up realises. I paid my dues in comfort eating. The thing is, the comfort only lasted as long as each mouthful, and on and off, I've gone through life dipping in and out of that safe habit place whenever the occasion arose, without quite knowing why I was there, or how to get back out again. Until this year when it all became clear.

At the time of writing this bit, I was a happily married busy career-type thirty-something. Two pregnancies made me a mother of two great kids, so now the fat's underneath a floppy belly and stretch marks. I'm a happy soul - most of the time, the food problem is always played down, right? Apart from the occasional domestic crisis, or when there was too much month left at the end of the money again. Just like with everyone else, overdraft-one, savings zero. Funny how each overdraft crisis was somehow temporarily cured with a chocolate biscuit or a bag of crisps. Still I sort of managed to get back down to a good weight for me – l0st 5lb - positively slim for me. Because - ah - let me recall. I was busy with my beloved, short-lived job as showbiz reporter on 'squarials' via BSB in 1990. Full timetable, empty belly, happy bunny.

But all good things come to an end (thanks Rupert), and the redundancies came, mine and my husband's, and then my Dad died, and then the new shopping channel job started. Shift work, perpetual mother's guilt, something missing at home, never-ending treadmill, not enough love and too much angst. I was a bit of a nervous wreck one Christmas – crying whilst wrapping the presents and then going in for my shifts at QVC - just 18 months after launch this fledgling shopping channel was doing well and I loved it. Plus I was strong, wasn't I? So without sharing my depression with anyone, I convinced myself the man wasn't having affairs, pulled my socks up, went back to the grindstone at work, suffered more mother's guilt, and had one too many all-inclusive holidays and the weight piled on.

My quest for the solution turned a major milestone when I came across the programme called Freedom Eating - The Seven Secrets of Slim People – in 1999 with guests Shawn and Vicky on QVC - & I haven't looked back since.

When the student is ready

Little did people realise it, but by the spring of 1999, I topped the scales at nearly thirteen stone - over 180lbs, and at 5'4"- that is not good. The scales don't lie. They hate you, but you can't ignore their self-righteous proclamation that you've been a gut-bucket. You know it anyway of course. I knew I'd been gaining at the rate or three or four lbs, every six months since I had my 'bit of a wreck' thing roughly four years before. Quite an impressive feat, to hide the lot beneath designer clothes. Ever bigger ones, admittedly. Holiday shopping at Easter and I couldn't even get into size sixteen white pedal pushers - oh bugger.

My first size eighteens.

A fitted, tailored TV wardrobe had always made it too easy to hide the extra inches. Slip into a tailored jacket as well as, thank you God, Lycra bootleg trousers, and voila! The acceptable shape of TV shopping - just. I swear if I wasn't constantly 'on-show', I'd have been a size 28 by that point. Acceptable until those keep-fit hours started to become less of a challenge and more of an occasion to get totally stressed out.

I really was well and truly overweight by now. In an hour of selling keep fit stuff, I'd do a few exercises, then get off and let the guest instructor 'show us all how you do the next bit'. Then one day I just couldn't push myself up on the incline-bench-pulley thing, made a joke out of it with lots of grunting and heaving and joking and laughing. *Ha-ha, funny fat lady*. But I felt bloody frustrated, and didn't my fellow presenter Paul make a meal out of it as only a skinny can! What could I do but join in? So they just did it more.

Fatty jokes had become a regular part of my repertoire, and I must say - the 10lb bars of chocolate we were selling, or the set of two rich, moist, fruit-cakes-in-a-tin, or the vertical roaster hours were crying out to be 'Debbie-fied'. Other show hosts mentioned my name in the same sentence as delicious food a little too often, and I began to truly start seeing myself as a 'fat person'.

-"I have to go easy with the butt toner - it takes three minutes for my backside to stop wobbling."

- "I'm just saving this crispy chicken skin for Debbie - I know she likes that."

- *"Now, to demonstrate this cleaner I've just made a big chocolatey mess on the carpet, good job Debbie's not around - she'd want to eat it."*

You know the routine, and I'll tell you more later. I must admit it was getting me down big time, and I knew I had to do something about it. But I love food - always have, and me and diets just never got on. I'd go on a diet, then come off a diet. I don't drink, smoke, gamble or a whole lot else and food was my panacea. The answer to everything. A crutch in good times and bad. You're lonely, you eat, you're angry, you eat, you're happy, let's go have a meal at the 'all-you-can eat' carvery and celebrate. "It's a special occasion, you eat, you can always go back on the diet tomorrow." "Yes," I'd think, "I might as well make the most of it tonight and stuff myself because tomorrow all this will be once more out of bounds." We've all done that, haven't we? I'd had more Last Suppers than normal dinners.

The roots were in my childhood, I know it, and so was the accompanying fear of deprivation, fear of being hungry - panic, in fact - at being hungry, instead of just realising that it's a normal body function and ties in with the hormones that control when to stop. But what did it matter what my body said? My brain told me it was time to eat. Lunchtime, break-time, anytime it was 'special' food, or 'free'. That's why the diets never worked. I already looked at food in a totally unnatural way anyway.

My mind chose limited, rationed and denied mode. I was constantly in deprivation and control

No chance my body would win through that lot. Let alone all those years of giving out messages of famine to my body by crash dieting, by always looking for the quick fix, making it lower my metabolism year on year with each diet. One of the most amazing facts discovered during learning Food Freedom for me was the study involving adults with normal appetites who were forced to go on diets. They actually automatically put on weight long-term as a result of consistently denying the body what it needed. Their metabolic rate had slowed down to accommodate this new situation of food sparseness, and they all had eating problems thereafter. The others who were given more food than they usually ate actually found their metabolisms also adjusted after a substantial time, and coped with all the extra food, and stayed higher thereafter.[1]

Being 'bad' is par for the course of a dieter's life, isn't it? And beating yourself up about it for the rest of the day is normal, isn't it? When the truth is, there's no 'good' or 'bad' behaviour surrounding food, there's 'just what the body wants,' 'what it doesn't want,' and crucially, *when* to eat it. And believe it or not, you can rediscover how to make use of this in order to get slim and stay there, whilst - amazingly - really having a good time enjoying your food and eating all your favourites whenever you're hungry. Unbelievable? Or achievable heaven?

Eureka

Imagine your food prison. You're in a big cage. No one knows it's there except you. The bars of this cage are the barriers that keep you from ever feeling 'normal' around food. You've been in this cage for so long, you think there is no key. The wrong rules keep you inside this prison. Do these still govern your life?

- *"You must finish your plate even if you feel stuffed."*

- *"You must have your vegetables then you can have some pudding."*

- *"You're too slow - eat faster."*

- *"You can't have cheese on top - it's fattening."*

- *"Look at your bum - it's cos of all those sweets you keep eating."*

-*"Don't have more bread - you won't eat your main course. "*

And so, so many more.

These rules help keep you in this prison. They are the bars through which you view the world and make your decisions surrounding every scrap of food that passes your lips. Now imagine someone comes along one day; a white knight on a charger, and declares that all these rules, which you've lived by for so long, inherited or made up for yourself, just... don't count. They aren't true, and you can ignore them. He unlocks the key to your prison and lets you out. *Oh my God. So this is where the slim people live!*

Want all those things you've been depriving yourself of for so long, all those things that skinnies have all the time - have them.

However, this is the crucial thing - the one condition - you only have it if your *body* really wants it. This book will help you distinguish those all important signals and tell you about the hormones our bodies use – and how for instance fructose in sugar can over-ride them. A calorie is truly not a calorie. (*Ed - *prophetic, given new studies in 2014*)

Also, it's actually fun learning the process and getting to know your body, your best friend, all over again.

It equally feels like heaven to say 'yes' to some of the foods you thought were 'bad' - but you're only saying yes to eating that one food, right there, right then, for as long as it feels good (not to a blow out 'cos you ate one biscuit too many!).

Or you might change your mind half way through and stop, because you can.

But what you're not doing is saying yes to losing control for the rest of the day, and opening the doors to a tidal wave of overeating because you've stepped outside the prison and all its rules. So eat it - without judgement - if you want it and that's the next crucial pointer. **You only eat it for so long as your body wants it.**

You stop when your body is satisfied, not when you can't breathe anymore. Not when you're full up. Just doing what the body would do naturally if your mind, and society, had never interfered. The body is magic, it knows these things.

And what a relief it is once you acknowledge that.

And what about all those times you "fill-up on vegetables." Well you don't have to, you know. Eat too much of any food and you'll put on weight. Eat at the wrong time, when you're not hungry, and your body will just put it into storage and convert it to fat. Eat loads of 'healthy' rice and vegetables all day long, then go to sleep and you can become a Sumo wrestler! Why do so many dieters feel they have to fill themselves up by overeating vegetables? They may be only vegetables, they are really, really good for you - but why overeat them?

There is an important point to be noted here, and that is that there are many people who trust themselves so little, that the mere thought of listening to the body to make food choices brings them out in a slight panic. If you're a serial dieter or if you just don't believe true food freedom can work for you, don't worry. There's a whole new section in the updated Till the Fat Lady Slims, out September 2014 just for you, if you feel safe around 'dieting', and want to ease yourself into all this freedom stuff gradually, then don't worry, you can. The most important thing is to feel comfortable and happy with it, and if you're too scared to go the whole hog immediately, then introduce it step by step - as recommended later in this book. But do it, if you can, even if you stay at step one for a year, because long term, it will be better for you than what's been happening in your life so far. Otherwise, why would you be reading this book? Don't be frightened. Yes, unlearning the beliefs you've had for donkeys' years will be a little scary at first, so give yourself permission to try it stage by stage, and enjoy the process. There are so many little exciting discoveries that make it all worthwhile. You just have to understand what they are.

Unlearning

Ever seen a baby turn its head and refuse to take any more bottle? It's had enough, and it stops eating. It just stops. You never force a baby to eat more, do you? Force the bottle back in its mouth? No! So why a toddler? Or a teenager, or an adult? If we hadn't been brain-washed over the years, throughout our childhood and adolescence and young adulthood and old adulthood, we'd never have lost that response. But it's not too late to get it back. Just think about it and you've got to admit it's true. We just need to unlearn all the 'manual over-rides' from years and years of deprivation and control.

Deprivation and control - yuk

Without deprivation and control, we'd be exactly how we were when we were born - with a specially evolved, perfect eating mechanism you can always trust to gauge exactly what to eat, and for how long, and when. It's called your body, and deep down within the confusion and desperation and fear, it's waiting. Just waiting to be handed back the keys to your mouth. Funnily enough, studies on babies' eating habits showed that even when some were fed on a more low-fat formula, their bodies automatically knew they needed to consume more, whilst they drank less if it was a richer concentration[1].

There is categorically no doubt that you *can* trust your body. Its inbuilt mechanisms for getting you what you need, when you need it, are lying dormant inside you, and what fun to bring them out of hibernation and into full use again! Make it fun - listen to your body-without judgement. Because judgement is the password to another Last Supper.

Pssssst! Hey, prisoner, here's an escape route for you - keep it to yourself though - only the skinnies know about this one! It's this: if you overeat one time, it's fine. 'What do you mean, fine? How can it possibly be fine? 'I've been bad.' No actually, skinnies will do what you call 'bad' things all the time. Want to be one of them? Well, how about this - just observe.

Don't judge.

Don't beat yourself up about it. If you want some chocolate - really genuinely want it, not in your head but in your body, have it. If you overeat a little, and pretty soon it'll only ever be a little, say to yourself - 'Interesting, I wonder why I did that,' and then just get on with your life. Don't waste any more time thinking about it, deliberating on what to do next, how to punish yourself for being such a terrible person, or generally being a food prisoner.

Act like a slim person- just move on.

Chapter Two –In the World of the Slim

The first steps to 'unlearning' all the beliefs that have made you fat...

There are certain facts that, once you discover them and accept that they relate to you, can really make you start to feel at home in this new world where the slim people live. Some times of the month, you may just need more food. Sometimes you may need less - in which case *don't* eat just because 'it's time to.' Or just because the family's about to eat. So? Just sit with them, with yours in front of you, and if you're not hungry, wait till you are and save it till later - why not? It's a good example to your kids too, if you need any more reasons! Later on when you're sufficiently hungry once more, it will taste better anyway. Then your body will be ready to digest, and not to store.

If you fancy a treat, pick your favourite food, the one that shouts at you - because that'll be your body telling you what nutrients it needs most at that time, if you listen carefully enough. And it won't always be the same! True - people who've always denied themselves certain things, for example, bacon, or raspberry milkshake, may find their bodies want *just* that for a while. But get enough and your body won't be shouting for it any more, and you'll move on from it. That's why, unlike with most diets, I'm going to say this - fill your house with your *most* favourite things.

Oh no, now she's really gone mad!

Are you thinking this – 'I know what I'm like if I have those foods in the house, I'll binge like, crazy, and once I've started I just can't stop' (remember can't = must). 'If I even think about those foods, or smell them, I start to get sweaty palms because I know they're my downfall....'

Well, hear me out on this one, ok? There's a defined logic to this argument, which you won't fail to understand, and as long as you follow it, and don't lose yourself repeating old habits - reliving your own history of overeating and reactions to foods - it will work.

If those 'danger foods' are there for the taking, your mind knows there's no shortage, and the craving for them will gradually go away. Tell yourself you can have one. Choose just that – eat it first – the next time you're hungry. Try it! Oh my God, it's a veritable gift from heaven that someone should even suggest this to you, but it's true. Say you can have it, really, really mean it. Say, "I can have it." Go on do it now, imagine that doughnut in your mouth. How lovely. "Oh yes, yes!" Meg Ryan's got nothing on you when this fabulous flavour fills your taste buds. Take another mouthful, then another, and keep observing what it tastes like – what it feels like in your mouth, as you swallow. Keep going until you get the deep breath, or until it doesn't taste as gobsmackingly wonderful anymore (and it will happen) then click in with the new decisions:

The New Decisions

- *"I don't have to finish it just because it's there."*

- *"I don't have to eat all of it."*

- *'I'm allowed to save the rest for later, and if I want it when I'm next hungry, I can have it all over again. But if I don't I won't."*

- *"If my body really, really wants more right now, I can have it."*

- *"If I'm not sure, I'll wait fifteen minutes, then assess it again."*

- *"I must just listen to my body and go with what it's telling me."*

- *"My body is giving me permission to go ahead and eat the forbidden foods, for a trade-off – I must take notice of it."*

- *"I will not let it down. In return, I will listen to the signals."*

Makes sense doesn't it? How many times do you eat things when you're on a diet that you wouldn't touch with a barge pole normally? It's just that if someone says you 'cannot' have the nicer versions, then it makes you want them more. Been there? Know the place? Bought the t-shirt? Food prisoners live in that place. Permanently. Remember that other important escape route. Say, "I can have it if my body really wants it, as much of it as I really want, till I physically don't want any more. Not till I'm full, or till they're all gone, or till someone comes in and sees me. Just till I'm "satisfied." Simple.

Liberation! Yes it is really possible to suddenly transform your life and not have to abide by those binding, restrictive, negative, depressing, straight-jacket beliefs you hear all the time - from yourself and others. It's a fabulous feeling, you wait till you try it.

Start listening to your body and not to your brain, or to anyone else's brain for that matter.

Then you'll be on your way to Food Freedom. If you always make your body eat diet food, even though it really wants just a little of the full-fat version, you'll probably feel totally deprived after eating the low-fat alternative, you'll go through the lot, and still come back to the 'bad' one in the end. Then feel that you've let yourself down again by 'giving in'. Think about the study using low-fat formula on babies. Hey, in life outside the prison, it's ok to have some of what you fancy - that old saying is never truer - but a little of what you fancy is almost certainly what you'll end up having if you allow your body to tell you when to stop. I'll say that again, because I've found it to be so true.

A little of what you fancy is almost certainly what you'll have if you listen to your body.

You only go into overdrive and finish the whole packet of chocolate chip cookies if your mind takes over and starts distorting your behaviour, you start feeling like a criminal for breaking 'The Rules'. If you can start to tell yourself it's all ok, and simply move on from each little misdemeanor, they'll be less and less frequent and that's what we want. After all, you're not going to get this perfect from the outset, and you can congratulate yourself because you are finally on a path to permanent weight loss.

Trust in your body - it knows what path to take. Your mind doesn't. It only thinks it does after years of being in the pilot's seat. It's just like flying an aircraft; 90% of the time, a plane is off-course, but every little correction brings it back on line till in the end, it's right on target[3]. That's what it'll be like when you start listening to your body and letting it do what it does naturally, without your mind interfering. But first you have to help it along. It doesn't happen overnight, but there are lots of little tips and extra guidelines to follow to help you give your body a chance to adjust. After all, you've been following these habits for years, right? So just like when you drive home and you go into automatic, and suddenly you've arrived, and you don't know how you got there? If you've followed that same route for years, it becomes ingrained in your psyche, biologically speaking: the electrical pathways in your brain are a well-trodden trail, and once you get going in the right direction, your body automatically takes over and knows which neuron connects to which and basically what to do next.

That's why you must be forgiving of yourself initially, whilst you scramble these old pathways, and take a refreshing new route at each key junction along the way. The more you get used to it, the more automatic the new way of eating will be in the end, and you'll be eating like a slim person. Establish new pathways and your mind will gradually let go of the old ones that made you fat. As it observes the transformation in your body, and in your being, and as you gradually shed the excess pounds left by overeating, your mind will learn to trust your body. You will instinctively know what you need to do, and more importantly than anything else, what you *don't* need to do.

Chapter Three - Ten Pounds of Lard

Don't let the scales decide if you're going to have a good day - throw them out!

Do you know how heavy ten pounds is? Ten one-pound packs of lard. Ten cans of soup. Put it in a carrier bag, walk up the stairs with it. Try to run with it. At the time of writing this chapter, November 1999, I've lost ten pounds of lard, and two inches off my waist. I've got more than twice that still to lose. How the hell did I get to be that heavy in the first place? It's still early days, but I've been adjusting to what's right for me using my new-found Food Freedom, and a useful kick-start I'll tell you about later. But, for the first time in my life, I'm confident and there's no reason to think the weight loss will stop. Sure there are ups and downs, but I'm sure as hell not going to punish myself for a hiccup in what amounts to a mere solitary measurement of progress – and one which doesn't give you the full picture. Yes I'm talking about that chief offender, the scales. The Food Freedom guide allows you to ignore the scales. I'll say it again.

Ignore the scales. Never get on them again. I said never!

You have full permission to go right ahead and walk straight by them. They no longer have the God-given right to set you up or knock you back for the rest of the day. They may cry out to be caressed by your 'plates of meat', but you shall fear not and resist their temptation because muscle is heavier than fat, and body weights fluctuate hour by hour, let alone day by day, so ignore them. The serial dieter weighs several times a day not just the once a week conventional wisdom recommends. What's the point of that? It's all just information in the end, but information doesn't change your life, unless you act on it, and incorporate it in a way that works for you. So ignore it, and as for the rest of the information that abounds and surrounds us in our daily fight against the flab, well, pick out what works for you and ignore the rest. **Begin Freedom Living too!** You should definitely follow your instincts and do what's right for you personally, using the guidelines given here, or in any of the Freedom Eating packs, or in the literature accompanying the numerous weight-loss clubs and magazines and books and videos and the rest.

I did, in fact, technically lose around seven pounds by counting points and doing Weight Watchers. They sent a lovely lady called Jacqui to me every week, with a fab supply of chewy breakfast bars, and caramel sweets and fruit pastille things that gave me the runs the day I over-ate them. Hang on a minute, did you say over-ate? Thought you didn't do that anymore.

Well, yes, I don't, now, but 'now' is Jan 2001. Oh yes time warp. Yes, I'm going back over my book, making additions, and I promised myself I'd include a little bit about Weight Watchers at this point. Just as a 'back to the future' type teaser, I can let you into a secret, I've now lost over two and a half stone - imagine how many pounds of lard that looks like! Anyway, more of what's to come in the next book, when I' ll tell you about what happened to me in the next year. Shall we say I've faced some major 'relationship challenges' and all the angst and comfort-eating that entails.

Then in September 1999, Weight Watchers offered to use me for PR purposes, and came to the QVC building in Battersea to sign me up to their program. The carrot for doing it was possibly featuring in one of their pieces in The Sun. Shallow and obvious, but the truth. So I followed it, and followed it ....till I couldn't stand it any more!

(Now I don't want to put off anyone from using slimming clubs if they really honestly work for you. Unlike the Freedom-Eating girls, I won't say 'never go', because I know a lot of people just don't ever think they can trust themselves enough to go it alone. You've been so used to getting guidance all your life that the mere thought of depending on your body's signals to choose what to eat, along with being given permission to eat all those things you've always thought of as 'forbidden', plus the idea of eating as much as you want, really blows your mind. If that's you, read this bit, but then make sure you read the bit later about combining with a diet plan. You just take the bits that work for you, and leave the rest out till you feel confident enough to tackle full on Freedom Eating).

Anyway, having started with gusto, I was gradually getting completely hacked off with the counting, the limitation, the 'can have, can't have' mentality. The 'lose half a pound = good girl, gain half a pound = bad girl'. Oh my God, we're talking about half a pound here. It descended to the farcical when I was asked, "have you had a poo yet, that could make a difference." Of course it would. Half a pound is ridiculous. I could put on half a pound and lose it again within a few hours. How can this be right, or good for me psychologically, to be measured by that and only that? Were we looking at percentage body fat? No. Even though there are some fab gadgets you can get nowadays if you really want to do this measuring lark. No, we were just weighing me. For goodness sake, at least give yourself a chance by not making weight loss the only consideration in whether you've been 'good' or 'bad'. Fat content may have gone down, even though your actual weight has gone up. Look at inches, even! I think every weight loss class in the country - no in the world - should be legally made to measure people by other factors, not just weight.

Anyway, so, needless to say, the morale starts taking a nose-dive, and pretty soon, I'm cheating on the 'what have I eaten this week' chart, I'm beating myself up all over again, having not done it for bloody ages. I'm exercising like a mad-woman to try to account for those couple of extra points I've consumed, and I'm driving everyone up the wall. Oh, and - just a minor point - I'm feeling depressed, obsessed, and stressed.

That's what conventional wisdom says is the 'way to go' to lose weight. Is it? Well you can keep it. The breaking point came at the end of October when we went away with the kids to a villa in Cyprus. Self-catering, so made the trip to the supermarket to scour the place for loads of non-fat stuff. Excruciating, for me and the man, and the kids - who had depressingly also started to act differently around food as a result of my obsessiveness again. Oh-oh. Danger. A couple of little secret binges and the old me started to re-emerge and I was frightened, and finally, turning into a rat-bag of the first degree was the last straw. I couldn't do it to myself, I couldn't do it to the kids and I couldn't do it to the man. So I made the decision to go back immediately to Full Scale Food Freedom, and by the time I got back home, Weight Watchers Jacqui was proud to announce that I'd actually lost a pound. Now had I stayed on WW, I'd have absolutely started bingeing and dieting, bingeing and dieting and would have gained the whole seven pounds back again, started making excuses why I couldn't make the weigh-in that week, and eventually given up, chiding myself for being a loser, a failure, and feeling ostracized from all the other goody-goodies who'd all lost weight that week but I hadn't. Sound familiar? It should. Apparently, the great majority - and it's been quoted at over 90% - of the weight lost through dieting and slimming clubs, is regained within a few years. So how can it work? Because 80% of the publicity for these places is generated by the 20% of the people who have lost, or are currently losing weight. We've all been privy to the conversations where our friends have boasted about that week's successful weigh-in. But do they often speak of the weeks where they put it on? No. The PR machine churns out success story after success story, prompting more and more troubled fatties to join up. But how many follow-up stories do we hear of? How many times do they revisit their champions from previous years? You get my point.

Now there are some exceptions to all this, maybe you're one of them - one of the few who have used a slimming club once to permanently lose weight, but the likelihood is that type of person hasn't spent a lifetime yo-yo dieting without success, and buggered up their metabolism completely in the process. Or quietly binged and felt so ashamed they daren't own up to anyone - including themselves. Often that type of person is a one-off dieter - and it works. If that isn't you, darling, and it certainly wasn't this fatty, well forget it! If you say, "but hang on a minute, Debbie, those clubs have always worked for me in the past, every time I go back there I always lose the weight." Hey, why the need to go back in the first place? It angers me because a fortune is spent treating the symptom and not the cause of weight gain. It's like trying to get someone to learn Chinese by showing them a pretty pattern on a page and telling them what sound to make when they see it, hey presto, you're 'speaking Chinese'. It works, till you forget what you were taught, become bored with the same old symbols, don't feel you're progressing, or just lapse back into speaking the same old language you're used to because you've done it for years.

If you don't understand what's underneath, it'll never be permanent. I tried to learn Greek once, with an audio tape and nothing visual. It lasted about as long as the holiday, but the French I got to know at school, and the German, even though I only did it for two years, sticks with me to a certain extent to this day because, we learned about what the verb was, how to conjugate it, what the genders are, how to use them, what the tenses are, and how they fit in. We understood it, so it stayed with us. And so it will be with Food Freedom. Once you understand it, you'll wonder how you lost touch with it for all those years. It's so easy, it's so bloody enjoyable, so logical, feels so good, you'll be hard-pressed not to go back to it time and time again, after every temptation to stray. Some people will never stray - it'll be as natural once more, as breathing. For others, like me, who live their lives on an improvement crusade, and are willing to go back to the hard work of finding other alternatives, going back to choosing with the brain not the body, listening to current thinking about various eating fads, or trying to abstain from certain foods, it'll be something to which you will always return with open arms at the end of a difficult journey, like coming back home at the end of the wars.

So diet if you must, but follow the early stages of Food Freedom at the same time, and you'll be well on the way to a more natural way of eating - the body's own way - the way we were born - the way our body wants to eat if we only give it the chance. Think, do I really want it? Does my body really want it? How will it feel afterwards? Do I really want more of it? Can I feel the food in my stomach yet? Stop if you can. And then gradually work towards trusting your own body once more. Give it back the control and you'll never need to suffer the indignities of being one of the 'bad girls' and feeling that old 'naughty little girl panic' as the slimming class begins to lose its shine once more.

Lecture over! Hehe!

So the seven pounds I lost on Weight Watchers I put down to counting. But you and I both know what would have normally happened at that point had I not gone back to food freedom. Another few weeks passed and I reached the ten pound stage. This was ten pounds lost since the initial WW weigh in, mind you, 12 st 6 lb. I have to say I was more than that originally, but I'd been scared to get on the scales for a long time. I'd not measured the loss in between starting Food Freedom and suffering the diversion of counting stuff, and going back to deprivation and control. But if you look at some of the photos, notably the one with Tony Robbins, the US Success Coach, when I hosted one of his hours in November 1998, you'd be shocked at the size of my face. And, bless his rapport techniques, even then he told me, "your husband's a lucky man." (If only he knew it, haha!). So having given up measuring, I couldn't be certain, but I know by appearance and past experience, I was over 13 stone - around 13st 4lb. I'd looked like it once before in my life - about the time of the spaghetti bolognese in the dustbin scenario - and I hated myself. Thank God for Food Freedom, it took me down to 12 st 6 lbs in around four months.

Chapter Four - Do What I Do

Water, and the body's many cries for help.

Okay, I own up. There are some things I'd like to recommend to you outside of the conventional Freedom Eating guidelines, and the first involves drinking water. Do it. There, I've said it. If I could get everyone to drink more water, even if it's just normal water, and not specialist ultra-hydrating versions, I'd be happy. But now I have to say you should do what feels right to you and your body, sure. But as far as water is concerned, just try it for a while for me and see! Yes, drink water, three litres a day is recommended, more accurately, drink half your body-weight measured in pounds, in ounces of water. For example, if you're 140lb (10 stone) then drink 70 ounces per day (16fl oz is about 500 ml). More and more is being discovered about how good it is to be fully hydrated. So I drank more water, and I exercised. I'm a firm believer in it, and if you are too, then great. But it's your decision you do what's right for you. The same thing goes with exercise.

Generally speaking, we all have known for years what we should be doing, and it's still the case. Don't get me wrong, what's best for your body is some exercise as well but you don't need to go mad! If you combine healthy eating with exercise, as many people do by just changing their lifestyle rather than treating it all as a temporary and drastic measure, you'll help yourself to stay younger longer, as well as helping your metabolism. We got a dog, (sorry Shawn, had to mention it!) in June 1999, and a good forty five minutes brisk walk every day has done wonders for my fitness and energy levels, my ability to walk upstairs without getting out of breath too much and my sense of well-being and being able to cope with those fitness hours on QVC once again!

Whatever exercise works for you, I personally recommend you do some, (check with your GP if you're unsure what type to go for), but walking, or a treadmill if you can't get out, is as good a place as any to start. Find something you enjoy, build it up gradually, but don't wear yourself out or give yourself a headache by doing too much too quickly and maybe you'll be able to feel little but consistent improvement over the weeks and months. Just get it into your life, somehow, even a few minutes a day, then build up from there. Again, listen to your body, and if it hurts, you're not doing it right! But exercise on its own is not the best way to use up the calories you've just eaten. You need to do half an hour's aerobic work-out to allow yourself a Mars Bar, or thereabouts, so you'd have to do some serious sweating or heavy physical work to balance out a typical huge eating binge. And any binge is by definition too much for your body's natural needs, so think seriously about the Food Freedom Guidelines and start practising Freedom Living if you also see life from inside an exercise prison.

How many people, especially guys, have you known, who believe the way to being slimmer is to work out all hours? Vikki Hansen's hubby used to work out, up to six hours a day in order to live life as a Grade A Gutbucket. He was fit not fat, but renowned for finishing off everyone else's leftovers, consuming mammoth portions and generally living in a different kind of prison - rules, rules, bloody rules. He believed that it would 'turn to fat' if he ever gave himself a breather and stopped the punishing exercise ritual. God forbid he should listen to his body's food needs and just maybe one day try not eating huge amounts.

If you live with someone like that in your life, then there's even more reason why this programme will be a Godsend. Imagine if he or she could stop and just consider the idea that they actually didn't have to maniacally stick to their training schedule if they just ate what their body wants and not what they think it wants. To not have to dutifully slave over a hot stepping machine for a couple of hours a day? Wow! It's liberation of a whole different kind.

I used to help my dad with his contract cleaning business whilst I was a student, oh yes, I've done my fair share of toilets, steps, supermarket floors, and corners and edges! And throughout that time, after a couple of hours of heavy labour, I remember still feeling guilty when I sat down with dad to a normal buttered, crusty roll come breakfast time. It felt forbidden to give my body food. All of it felt forbidden. The only way I could conceive of it being 'good' was if it was slimming bread or crackers with slimming spread and a scraping of marmite or a dry, boiled egg. And should I ever dare to transgress, especially that early in the day, and step into the World of Forbidden Food, then I really had to go the whole hog. Should I have that little chocolate bar as well... or not? A chocolate bar for breakfast? Not a chance nowadays. Yuk, but it was deliciously bad back then, as I devoured it and sometimes went back for seconds - again, which my body didn't want, but my brain wanted.

All to make the most of being in the Forbidden Zone before being locked up again.

Nowadays breakfast is a simple affair. I know what I need first thing, at the time of writing – 2000 - a cup of tea (decaf or herbal when I'm in the mood, but mostly basic Tetley!), and a couple of Rich Tea biscuits. Heaven. And nowadays, I don't have to spend the rest of the day feeling like I've started off on the 'wrong' foot, and consciously cutting down to make up for it, or ending up blowing the lot because I've started off badly.

They say breakfast is the most important meal of the day, well yes, for some people it can be, but hey, guess what, try drinking a big glass of water before you even begin contemplating what to eat, and see what a difference it makes to the way your head feels fifteen minutes later. My guess is, if you're anything like I was, you'll possibly even feel a little sick first thing in the morning due to being dehydrated, muggy headed, sluggish, and lethargic, your pillow feeling like a magnet. What your body's signals may be trying to tell you, and your brain is misinterpreting, is that you need water, not food or coffee. Many diets make you feel better because they recommend upping your water intake, and it's the resulting hydration that makes you feel like it's working for you, not necessarily the strict diet regime. Think again if you ever catch yourself saying, "but I feel so healthy when I'm on that diet." It may be just the extra water. (And of course more fresh produce is going to help your body because it's mostly water too, as well as valuable roughage!) There's nothing like a good clear-out! And since a 'clear-out' needs water to help it on its way, no wonder many of us live our lives permanently constipated if we spend the day drinking nothing but diuretics like tea and coffee. At least balance it out by having extra water.

Drink as much water as you can reasonably do.

If you really feel like a coffee, then fine, but this brings me on to another Secret Escape Route - listen to your body and find out what's a good fit. Sometimes you can end up with a headache if you combine a coffee with a doughnut first thing in the morning, whereas if you drank the coffee, with water maybe and waited till you were sure you were genuinely hungry, body hungry, for a doughnut, then it may be perfectly ok. Or perhaps you'll need to leave the coffee till a little later in the day, or have it with two glasses of water, or black, or decaffeinated. Or change the brand as a different one may not give you a headache at any time of day. Certain combinations of food might not work for you. Perceived wisdom nowadays about food-combining means keep proteins away from carbs and you might be ok, less bloated and so on. Everyone's saying don't have so much white bread, pastas and so on. Well, hey, your body might just agree with them! But if it does, it's not like someone else telling you what to do, it's your own flesh and blood, literally giving you signs that something is working. Or not. And all you have to do is listen. Just listen to your body every time and you won't go far wrong.

Then, you make the leap to complete Food Freedom, once you allow yourself to acknowledge a luxury - that no food takes you into the psychological Forbidden Zone. Nothing does. Ever. So you're less and less likely to fail, each time you do this. Less likely to end up repeating the bad patterns of the past. Once you know you can have it, you think about it differently. Therefore you allow yourself to consider if you actually really want that flavour in your mouth right then. Maybe you won't, ever again. Maybe some days you will, some you won't. Maybe you will till your body starts to realise that this new found Food Freedom is not just some passing fad, just like all those others have been in the past. It's for real, and it's here to stay. And you really could have cheesecake for lunch, dinner and supper if you genuinely wanted it. Body hungry, remember? (NB – you wouldn’t – not for long. That’s why it works. It just ceases to be ‘treasure’ any more). Then you're less likely to be in 'famine' mode, and more likely to be transforming yourself into a person no longer frightened around food, scared of being let off the leash because you can't trust yourself to be 'good'. Oh my God, it's so life-changing, this whole Food Freedom process.

I so want to give this gift to other people, and you will too - you'll want this new-found freedom for your nearest and dearest the same way I want it for mine. And do they all listen and are they all converted? Nope. Do they hell....

Chapter Five - Suffering the Slings and Arrows

You don't have to be fat to have a food problem.

People are always cynical, aren't they? It's normal for a socially conditioned adult in this day and age to doubt some raving loony who declares they can eat what they want from now on. They will always try to doubt you, but just wait, keep doing what you're doing, and the proof of the pudding will be in the - well the *not* eating, and the new shape they'll gradually see appear on you, and the happiness and liberation you'll exude.

They will try to inflict their conditioning back on you - oh, expect it - like the girl at work, size eight, food-obsessed Jane, who said to me once I'd started to lose weight, and was comfortably indulging in half a Danish pastry one lunchtime, "should you be eating that if you're on the telly?"

Like my mum, who, before she got used to the idea of my Food Freedom used to repeat the same old statements of my childhood - "don't eat that, you'll put all that weight you've lost back on again." God, the temptation to let anger swell up and have a row, but guess who's already the winner here? It's not them. Just smile sweetly and carry on eating it. That'll get their goat more than answering back ever would. Or say, "when I chose to eat it, I didn't have you in mind." Hee hee! Give it time, and they'll want to know more about how you've done it, and that's the time to tell them more. *When the student is ready, and all that, and you're ready right now, or you wouldn't be reading this*. Even if you only do the first few stages, and leave the more daunting stuff till a later date, you're ready. Probably more ready than you've ever been in your life, and so fed up of being on the same old yo-yo treadmill; one that has so many rules you don't know where to begin. Well start by just not beating yourself up and considering yourself 'bad' if you stray, especially first thing in the morning.

So for me, a cup of tea and a biscuit about half an hour after I'd woken up and drunk lots of water was ideal. But for years before that, I'd tell myself off if I started the day like that. And a telling off at the start of the day was a sure fire way to end the day full of remorse, self-disgust, and self-pity, as well as having consumed far too many calories, all of which my bloody brain told my body to eat, because I'd started off 'bad'. So I was in the 'bad zone' and could carry on acting that way, and feeling like shit as a result, and overeating to try to feel better, which it did, the moment the food was in my mouth. But then the guilt came back, and the pattern continued. Overeating, comfort eating, stress eating and just... eating. And I could have broken it at any time by just being a witness not a judge, preventing more bad feeling leading to more overeating. All because my brain told me to. Even though, ironically, my body would have been happy with a fraction of that food.

Because from somewhere in the distant past, my body remembered being the one who made the decisions on what it actually needed in that instant – which food, just water, or maybe absolutely nothing. But once our brains kicked in and started over-ruling, we were on the pathway to obesity, we just didn't know it yet.

In fact, once the kids were born and I was at home looking after a toddler and a baby, I rarely ate at breakfast time, because I knew if I succumbed to something I perceived to be 'bad', and went down that route, I'd end up stuffing myself with all the wrong things by late afternoon. So I missed breakfast and starved myself thinking I was being' good'. So by the time I'd gone way past hunger and was actually starving, my poor body was craving everything in sight. Another Secret Escape Route is don't go past hunger to being starving or you won't be able to hear your body's signals that it's reached satisfaction. The first few times you'll probably misjudge it anyway, and eat a little too much that time, or stop too early and need to eat again fifteen minutes later. Just remember the flying the plane analogy, it's off course for 90% of the time till the pilot makes a little correction then it's back on course again, and that's how learning Food Freedom is.

Don't judge and don't be the critic, just observe and move on.

I did find however, pre-30 years old, that being busy helped to keep my 'problem' under wraps. Plus, before the big three-O, a couple of weeks 'cutting down' and I'd go back down to about 10st 5lb, no trouble. That may sound heavy to some people, but I've got a lovely photo of me at that time in some jeans I've kept for posterity, the idea being one day I'd get into them again. The fateful one day we all dream of. We all buy clothes specially for it, which sit in the back of the wardrobe unworn, labels intact. But thanks to Food Freedom, it's now in sight, at the end of a shorter, brighter tunnel, and what *your* ideal weight is, is just another whole category of 'rules' just waiting to be broken. You aren't going to be a Kate Moss or a Michelle Pfeiffer if your body doesn't naturally want to go there. Settle for being happy and content, and living a life outside the Food Prison and you won't end up caring what your weight is. It's whatever is natural for you once you start giving your body a chance to do the decision making.

Remember, ignore the scales.

Some of you may remember the dreadful days of Twiggy being the role model to all impressionable young females around the world. Well if you were naturally shaped like a Jayne Mansfield or a Marilyn Monroe, tough. Maybe that was where your problems really started, at school or in your later, still formative years, when other people's opinions mattered so much to you it made you change your way of life, and beliefs about yourself in order to try to conform to their ideals? Think of Cliff Richard, the Perennial Peter Pan of British Pop. He was an upcoming young pop star in the early sixties when he heard a character on a new soap opera, Coronation Street, saying, "that tubby Cliff Richard," or something like that, and it affected him big-time, making him diet to lose the chubbiness. Is that what first started you out being a serial dieter because someone in their wisdom somewhere said you were fat? Or round? Or 'pleasantly plump', or some such throw-away remark, never realising how appalled you were and how it changed you - forever, in some cases.

Until now. Was it a parent, with their well-meaning, or sometimes not so well-meaning comments, said in the hope of connecting your behaviour because it just didn't fit in with their ideals? The never-ending family chants:

- *"Don't eat that, or your bum'll get even bigger."*

- *"Should you be eating that with a shape like yours?"*

- *"Do you think dessert is a good idea when your holiday is coming up."*

- *"You'll never get into your bikini when we're away if you keep on eating bags of crisps all the time."*

They're blatant. Equally dangerous, but not so obvious, are the subtle ones, the ones that we all tell ourselves are common sense, especially when dealing with children.

- *"Don't eat those now, you won't eat your dinner."*

- *"Don't eat dessert before your main course."*

- *"Eat your greens and you'll get dessert."*

- *"You must clean your plate, just think of all those starving children in Africa/China/ Romania."*

- *"Don't leave your crusts."*

- *"Don't eat too many, only have one or two or you'll spoil your dinner."*

Now these may be more acceptable to our way of thinking nowadays. After all, we're not 'good parents' if we don't control our children's diets, and teach them to eat well, are we? Hmmm, 'good parents / bad parents', now where have we heard this sort of dichotomy before? Think it through. We drum it into our kids that they can't be trusted to get it right. If they start believing they shouldn't trust themselves where food's concerned, it means we're implying that they can't trust their bodies. What chance do they stand of developing natural eating as they get older? We see it all over the Western world nowadays in childhood obesity, fat kids who've unlearned how to eat perfectly for their body's needs, and are now sadly eating for other reasons, and very often it's to please their parents. Ever been subject to this one?

- *"Look, she's finished her plate, haven't you done well?"*

- *"Been really good, eaten everything."*

- *"You've done well eating all that restaurant meal."*

Why is overeating in a different place 'doing well'? A throwback to the days of rationing I reckon, and a knock-on effect we could do without. So stop it, and spare your kids the next cycle. A little girl I know called Sam is like this. She's renowned for eating everything on her, and sometimes her brother's plate. She is always on the lookout for food, like an animal on the prowl, always asking for more, always acting up if she doesn't get it, or doesn't get enough. She's not fat now and her mum is actually fairly skinny, but her mum has a big food problem. **You don't have to be fat to have a food problem.**

How many of us hear a slim woman complain about her weight. "You must be joking," we think. "You've got to be kidding. This is fat!? I'd love to look like you!" But if a person feels it, then it's true for them, and it means they've got a food problem. If their lives revolve around food, even size eight Jane at work who's obsessed with her, and everyone else's, shape. Poor cow. I'd finished the rest of that Danish with a smile on my face and a glee in my heart that I was free! Whilst she, as slim as she was, was very definitely still locked up, and the extent of her obsession, even having to watch other people's weight for them, probably means she'll never get out. And one day she'll be fat and forty and completely caught up in the whole yo-yo thing. Just wait till she has kids. Poor kids.

It's just a matter of upbringing, or background, or experiences in life that lead us to develop our current belief systems, and it's really heartbreaking that so many kids have parents who start interfering with how they would naturally eat so soon after learning to talk. Let's be honest here. Remember the baby bottle story? We wouldn't dream of forcing the rest of a bottle of formula down a baby's neck when it's firmly clamping its mouth shut and turning its head away. But as soon as the kid can understand us, we're forcing it to finish bigger quantities of food than it really needs, by saying, "eat all your dinner," and to ignore their naturally quiet whisper of satisfaction. We're demanding that to fit in with our social conditioning, and the tribe's expectations, that they consume foods they don't necessarily feel like, right then and there, using blackmail or bribery to achieve our goal. Ignoring the fact that they may well feel like exactly that if you let them wait a bit longer. Or to just naturally graze a little instead of making them sit down to a complete meal because it suits you, and worse, to chastise them when they don't conform. What's the message, for God's sake? Don't trust your body. Trust me.

Like the snake from The Jungle Book, a parent has the hypnotic effect that starts the unlearning process at an early age. One of the biggest favours you could do a child is to let them eat when they're hungry, allow them to pick and choose at will. It's not good to make them wait for meals. If their little bodies are hungry now, they're bloody hungry now. Just because it doesn't fit in with your plans for mealtime, so what? Importantly, don't use sweets as reward or offer snacks in between meals and make sure what they're offered for dinner is tasty and wholesome and you're enjoying it too. Why give a kid nuggets chips and beans if you're having a tasty stir fry?

Surely a happy, satisfied youngster is more important than you getting your way about mealtime. Give a little, and adapt. I'm not saying let them eat sweets and no dinner ever, and I'm not saying this is the solution for every child out there. But I am saying just find a compromise to help them off this vicious spiral that may end up in them emulating you in adulthood. Would you really wish that on someone you love? Well it's early enough to make a change right now. If I can, you can, believe me. I did last summer with my own two, aged then, twelve and nine.

At May half-term, when I first began to lay-off Lauren and Brad, and broke the patterns I'd had when I was a kid, and not say a word about what or when or how to eat, amazing things started to happen. Just as I began leaving the food on my plate, and not coming out with so many learned 'rules' about food, mealtimes, quantities and so on. Just as I became less and less strict with my own eating, so Brad began to lose the puppy fat he'd gained so distinctly two summers before.

Bless his little heart, he'd been the top athlete in year five at the school sports, but a year later, he'd gained a little too much weight, his face was very full and round, his trousers began not to fasten. He wasn't fat, but he wasn't that naturally slim, like the boy he'd been before. Maybe it was a knock on effect from the tough time I was giving myself at that point, or from the stresses my marriage had been going through, or maybe he was stressed about school, who knows. But he was beaten by the boys in the year below in those key races at his final school sports that summer, when everyone else expected him to win, and my heart went out to him. But what was my family's reaction? "That's because you've put on weight, Brad. If you hadn't eaten all those sweets and crisps this year, you would have won." Poor little sod. Need I say more about the effect this then had? It was also then followed by that house move away from everything he knew, too. No wonder he was having a little bit of a problem getting into his new grammar school trousers. Until Food Freedom.

Thank God for Freedom Eating.

It's one thing when it affects your own life, but quite another when it impacts so profoundly on those so fundamentally important to you, like your son. Thank you, Vikki and Shawn, for giving me this freedom. I only hope it can help others in the same way, and it's so easy to do too. Needless to say, with the relaxing of my attitude, as well as being at that age where they start to sprout up, he'd slimmed right down by the end of that summer. Proud or what! It may have happened a bit naturally, anyway, but I knew I'd helped. My husband Tony, however, came with a whole host of different rules about eating. He had slings and arrows of his own, just a different kind.

Chapter Six - A Partner in Crime

The perils of contentment.

"She's content, that's why she's put on weight.... He's happily married, we all know what that does to a man." Beer bellies and bigger dresses. The effect our partner can have on us is the next big strain in the unlearning process.

Seeking approval is, possibly, the biggest fundamental mistake we ever make throughout our lives. Wayne Dyer says, "Be independent of the good – and bad - opinion of others."(4) Sound advice. If only we could do it with those we love the most. Maybe you went through your childhood absolutely ok. I know a girl who grew up on a farm and had enough daily physical activity to counteract a grown man's calories. She was absolutely fine till she left home at seventeen and got comfortable with a man who loved his food and had a tendency to overeat. It's amazing how quickly we can start to override our bodies' natural signals. She then put on weight and shared his problems with food.

But don't forget should it happen to you, with a new partner, in the midst of all these new intentions, it's just as easy to bring yourself back to Food Freedom again – gently and kindly. And then once the kids come along, your own comments to them may be sorted, but perhaps it's your partner that's now being the Food Nag.

My own husband's problems had to be addressed too, as they obviously also had an impact on how our kids ate. My hubby's a slim person. He used to be a skinny but he's never in his life been 'fat'. He's 'one of them'. Mrs. Food Problem marries a partner who hasn't got a clue about permanent overeating. He's never done it. His mum was, and still is, one of those who would serve the most delicious foods, but always in small quantities. When I first started to eat with them, I always came away feeling secretly deprived, I suppose because I felt the helpings hadn't been big enough. Oh, I was satisfied, all right, her portions weren't always far off what it would take to make an adult satisfied, roughly a fistful of food, (rough guide only) but my beliefs over-rode my body and I went off to stuff cakes and biscuits afterwards.

She also made lovely cakes for her family, and they all used to eat them and not feel so guilty that then they over ate in secret later.

Sometimes, as a skinny, Tony would polish off a whole tin of little cakes, or pack of biscuits, but - and it's a big but - he wouldn't beat himself up about it, and then go through the rest of the cupboard to eat loads more because he felt bad. He might have felt uncomfortable, and that's why he didn't do it again for a while. And more importantly, he'd eat less later. And he didn't play the mental tennis a food prisoner plays every time they binge.

As a parent, Tony did however, come out with the more subtle 'common sense rules' about meals and eating. These were indeed heavily drummed into him as a child, as well as a whole host of others I never had - about cutlery and elbows and talking and always leaving a little - and the list goes on. The so-called 'polite' rules about food and mealtimes, which were the legacy of his father and mother. If this works for you, then great. But we just knew we had to ease up on all the rules to make this work for our kids. And it paid off big-time.

He was always a slim-Jim at school, and through his teens, and into his twenties. When we first met, and for sometime afterwards, I'd be heavier than him. Not a bad achievement considering I'm 5'4" and he's six foot tall. To some extent his 'don't care' food-attitude helped me be less obsessed too. You do pick up other people's behaviour traits if you're around them often enough. And in my leaner years, before our troubles kicked in, I'd find it easier to say 'no' if he did too, to that extra square of chocolate, or that second slice of cheesecake. But having been an accomplished 'secret food criminal', the underlying habits were only in remission rather than gone forever. Tony would eat biscuits like there was no tomorrow sometimes, and cakes like they were going out of fashion - if they were his favourites. He always ate what he most liked (one of the key Secrets of Slim People), and then, out of nowhere, he'd be able to stop - just like that. He could almost always just say no to extra helpings, and dessert, anathema to me at the time, especially after a slap-up meal in a nice restaurant. Special occasion = become gutbucket. Enter Forbidden Zone. Abandon all vestiges of normal eating and fill body with food. Why are the 'eat all you can' menus so popular in restaurants? Because for most of us, we're a nation of food prisoners.

Now I know that you don't have to be a sheep as far as restaurants are concerned. You can be a free-thinking individual who asks for extra mayo on the side, and orders dessert to come at the same time as main course, and – shock, horror! - even eats dessert first if that's what you're most in the mood for. And then, in the spirit of stopping at satisfaction, and if you don't like waste at least keep a bit of it for later. And by stopping earlier on the main course, you can reserve a little bit of space in your belly so you can fit in a little something sweet, if you know you'll want it. But it's probably going to be a LITTLE bit, given you're probably not far off satisfied after eating dinner first!

It's just a matter of planning ahead. This means stop eating the main course before you reach satisfaction, knowing you'll take the remainder home. Great Secret. Remember, you can almost always take the rest of the meal home in a 'to-go' box, most restaurants do them nowadays. Isn't it better to take it home rather than stick it down your neck at a point when your body isn't able to deal with it, and therefore has to store it and therefore make more fat? Most restaurants get asked for a takeaway box or 'doggy bag' all the time, and after you've done it a few times, you'll be used to it too. And so will the people you're with. They'll stop commenting as they see you gradually start to lose weight. One thing most people notice of a fatty is if they finish their plate or not. They'll be proud of you, and more importantly, you'll be proud of you as you push the barriers back and face successive challenges in your mission to escape permanently from Food Prison, and leave stuff on your plate. Enlist their help if they ask you about it, and they'll possibly even feel like doing it themselves sooner than you or they would have expected.

It'll certainly at least be refreshing to have someone around them who is free of the shackles of food prison, illuminating the way to a much nicer land, a free place, where there are no restrictions from your brain about what type of food you eat. It's such a pleasure to eat with Food Freedom, where every option is judged the natural way, the way it would have been had we never meddled with our body's control mechanisms. If you have any problem with this, it is usually all about convention. Well, buck the system! Don't kowtow to other people's ideas of what you should do, or to your partner's. It feels so fantastic to feel one-upmanship over a skinny beautiful woman, size eight Jane for instance. Oh, I forgot to tell you, the Danish pastry episode was after I'd already let go the fact that she'd secretly put sweetener in my tea instead of the sugar I'd asked for! Buck the system. Speak up for yourself if you want to too, if you can't make yourself ignore their comments with a smile. Like I did with Jane.

"Do you know," I said, a warm fuzzy feeling pervading through me, "this is precisely how I have been losing weight, over ten pounds now, believe it or not." And then I smiled in a way she knew I meant it and left, knowing she couldn't quite fathom how it was possible. As I said, now *there's* a girl with major hang-ups about food. She's a chubba-lubba waiting to happen. Because with beliefs so strong she even wants other people to obey the rules she lives by, it'll only be a matter of time before one day, the rules get the better of her, and she caves in and stuffs herself as a way of life. Over and over again, till she gets fat. She's a fat person in a skinny's body. It's a novel concept, but I believe it's true. She may look great, but she's bloody miserable, and more than that, she doesn't enjoy her food. Mealtimes are probably just as much a nightmare to her as to you and originally to me. So one day she'll burgeon.

Hate to say it, but it was far too much self-righteousness for me. I mean, fancy even secretly deciding I shouldn't have sugar in my tea! Poor girl, quite funny really. Know someone like that? Well next time, things will be different. I promise you. Just give Food Freedom a go, and your whole life will change. And once you start Freedom Living, you'll never want to live any other way again. For instance, have a starter as your main meal. With extra side orders if you want. Or just have a few side orders as your meal. Check in with your body and see what jumps out at you from the selection on offer, and if you're not sure, why not order both and see what then tastes the best, because that's what your body will be needing: whatever tasted the best. So eat that till you're satisfied, and take the rest home. And never be afraid to ask to share a single portion, especially in places where one dish is enough for two, and especially when you've let the waiter know you'll look after them so they don't mind serving less food if their tip is not based on the total bill. If there's any food left, start as you mean to go on and always ask for a doggy bag.

Break down the barriers in your life! Do it, in front of everyone! Especially if that dish was so delicious you'd like to repeat the experience later on at home, why waste it once you're past satisfied and it just doesn't taste so good any more? And what's more, you are now officially totally freed from the necessity to do the opposite, and finish off other people's portions! Or 'eat it just because it's there.' Or mum cooked it specially, or the kids left it or I haven't got a container to take it home in and it's expensive...

They are all reasons your mind suggests to override your body's needs and requirements, but you don't have to live that way anymore!

Sure sometimes, something may be so delicious you just feel like eating a little too much of it. But satisfied means not being able to feel the food in your stomach even a little bit, and if you can, but it was worth it, because it was just so enjoyable, guess what, you're not going back to prison! You have been given an official perpetual 'Get Out of Jail Free' card valid for the rest of your life. So don't forget you always theoretically carry it, and can use it whenever you need to, in order to remind yourself you don't behave like that anymore. Yes you truly don't behave like that anymore and the great news is, this can apply to partners too. I don't think I've ever known The Man to be hung up on what he's eaten. On what he's drunk, maybe, but that's another story!!

What a weird unimaginable way to live your life, not being hung up on food!

I always thought it was inconceivable that someone could actually walk away from mints on the table at the end of a meal. Wasn't it part of some unwritten code that you simply have to eat them all? And also eat anyone else's left lying around? Why not just fill your home with your favourite after dinner chocolate mints and then they won't hold such a fascination if you allow yourself them on a regular basis. You won't really want many, either.

Christmas Dinner was another big occasion for a blowout of enormous proportions. Why does everyone do it? If we did it all year round, it wouldn't have 'scarce' attached to it, and come December 25th, maybe we could reach the Queen's Speech at 3pm without feeling like our stomachs were going to explode, and being unable to do anything except sit in a corner snoring and dribbling for an hour amidst wrapping paper, toys with run-down batteries and nut shells.

And another thing. As a natural ‘skinny’, The Man could actually go to watch a film and not want popcorn! What? Sometimes I'd go to the pictures just to eat the popcorn! Nowadays, I'd eat it before the film, so that I followed another Secret Escape Route from Food Prison.(5) Don't do anything else at the same time, so you can enjoy the food to its fullest, and not feel at the end that someone else must have sneaked up and scoffed some because you don't remember eating that much! And nowadays I'd take the popcorn home if I had any left, after buying a much smaller portion than I used to anyway. Or just leave it. Gasp, shock horror!

Chapter Seven - Ecstasy on a Plate

For food lovers everywhere - how to get the most out of your meal.

Do you know what? The best thing you can do to achieve Food Freedom, is don't do anything else whilst eating. This helping hint has been one of the most instrumental in letting me understand my body – why? Because you can hear its signals. It's also one of the easiest things you can do as a first step. The first change, to eating your way into Freedom gradually.

Particularly if you feel you can't let go of a diet plan or you're already going to a slimming club or whatever. Just do the basics first, and then afterwards you can work your way up to full Food Freedom gradually. When I started doing the Freedom Eating system, around May 1999, this was the part which took the most effort. I'd always done more than one thing at once, even down to watching the TV and reading at the same time. It used to infuriate the hell out of hubby Tony. Maybe being on constant open earpiece for my TV work made this an automatic habit, talking and listening, (sometimes to a much more interesting conversation than you were having yourself live on air!). At the start of Freedom Eating, I found it all so fulfilling and rewarding, I actually soon found myself WANTING to sit out in the kitchen and eat on my own, instead of taking food into the lounge. Now the family rarely eat in front off the telly. It helps to keep the cream sofa clean too, mind you! But a by-product of this is that we're having family meals around a table together, which is great for communication and a bit of 'us' time.

Don't do anything else whilst eating.

I also used to find it a bit infuriating when Tony didn't take advantage of the Help-Yourself-Salad Bar like all my lot did. Ah, yes, the Pizza Hut help yourself salad bar. I remember it well. I was the expert in standing the cucumber up around the edges of the bowl to make it deeper, so I could stack the plate up higher, then eat the lot before the pizza arrived. And I won't even begin to tell you about that self-service holiday at Pontins. Or the as-much-as-you-can-eat Chinese meals we had. No wonder our family nearly all have a tendency to chunkiness! The embarrassment of walking back through the restaurant with a huge plateful was far outweighed by the feeling of victory in my bones as a result of greedy-pig tactics. But family rules and habits are some of the hardest to break, aren't they? Being the eldest of five kids – seven in our family in total - had its advantages when it came to getting my share of treats. For instance the packets of cakes which came in fives. After mum and dad had gone shopping on Friday each week, all hell let loose. If you didn't get yours early, you wouldn't get it at all. So you ate it whether you were hungry or not! So everything basically as gone by Monday, and the rest of the week we were all constantly on the lookout for extras. If I'd known what I know now, if someone had just told me all this then, I would have found everything so much easier to cope with. I'd have found life easier to cope with!

After all, the signs of gluttony were there even in the early days.

Early warning signs

One of the earliest memories relating to food was once I'd reached about ten. The slightly tubby young Debbie Flint was featured, in a picture with the other kids from the Wandgas Cricket Club on our first proper holiday away together, to Warner's in Hayling Island. It was fab. Left to our own devices more or less the whole week, meals at our own pace with the parents safely tucked away in bars or around the pool, and I thought I was the bees knees in that short yellow dress. Let alone the little top and beige hot pants. But when the photos came back I made up my mind to start watching my weight - like mummy did. So bang went my final memory of being slim. From then on, I classed myself as one of the fatties. I wasn't, of course. But the inevitable classroom comparisons between the cuddly, the slim and the downright skinny girls didn't help. Later on, neither did the vicious self-consciousness of being a teenager – giving rise to an evil division between those of us who were regarded as fat, and those who were thin. The thin ones could fit into all the latest suede skirts and halter tops from Chelsea Girl, and hot pants were par for the course. But my noticeable pudgy bits inside the tops of my thighs were the bane of my life in those pre-midi skirt days, and soon, sure enough, I began to feel guilt surrounding food. I started to diet, at age twelve.

Exercising all that deprivation and control was all my mind needed to tip me over the edge. No more balance. The spiral had begun. Thing is, I did manage to get a little slimmer over the course of the next two years. And by the time I left Morden Farm Middle School in Merton, SW London, I considered myself a seasoned dieter. My first grown up clothes for high school from Martin Ford in Sutton were slimming and fashionable. But little did I expect that by the next Christmas, they wouldn't fit me. If I'd known that diets don't work, it never would have happened.

There was some element of being 'grown-up' if you had to watch what you ate, wasn't there? All the 'it' girls were on diets, weren't they? And you could easily do it, even at school, if you had the determination and drive. Back at middle school, I'd just skip lunch and sit outside getting more and more starving. We'd learned that no one realised or checked up once you were in the top year. So we starved ourselves, in front of each other, but got progressively hungry as the long afternoon wore on. More than ready by the end of school to get home and immediately wolf down about four slices of marmalade on toast, in private, on my own. Then also have dinner later. I always ate it because mum expected me to. It was completely alien to leave it. In later years I'd even have two evening meals, one at the boyfriend's and then one back at mine when he dropped me off, because we'd forgotten to tell my mum we'd eat at his, or vice versa. Overload city. But at least I didn't get told off.

But I firmly believe having delicious school dinners was at the crux of the first true food problem I ever had, and loving food like I did, and with an inherited set of rules like I had, what chance did I stand? What chance did any of us stand? I'd always loved the school dinners - ours were heaven at Morden Farm Middle School with the on-site kitchens and amazing cooks. I have never since tasted such bliss in a custard pot.

Prior to the skipping meals season, I'd regularly finish up any extras left by the skinnies on our school dinner table at lunchtime. Already my brain had forgotten how to do 'satisfied'. Already I had discovered the Forbidden Zone, and camped out there every dinner break. How much was I in my element if it was a dinner which my schoolmates and juniors on my table, didn't like? And who fought hardest to be 'monitor', on the table with the 'emaciated' first years who never liked the skin on the custard? All the more for me! Oh my God, I remember being in rapture at meal times in those days. Thing is, unbeknown to me, those little skinnies were also in rapture, they just knew when to stop.

The Queen's Jubilee in 1977 also stands out in my mind. By now I was fifteen, and should have known better. Our street was having our party in the school hall. The night before, all the packets of cakes, biscuits and sweets were all delivered to the stage, and sat lined up in row after row of stodgy indulgence, a silent witness to our great nation's need to eat crap at times of celebration. Everyone had gone home, and as my dad was the school caretaker, I sneaked back in, supposedly to find him. I crept into the darkened hall, heart pounding - a mixture of terror and anticipation that in just a few minutes, a precious stolen few of those illicit goodies would be mine. I made my way up to the stage, and surrounded by an almost tangible feeling of awe and excitement, started to search through the bags for my best choice of booty. Chocolate Snowballs or Wagon Wheels? 'Everyone's a fluffy one' marshmallow biscuits or Cadbury' s fingers. I tried to take from bags where it wouldn't be noticed, no one would have kept a record of what went where, surely? I knew there was far too much food for the party, and tried to reason with myself that it was ok, it was my right to steal away some of these forbidden fruits long before anyone else had the chance to get at them. How I thought it was my right, God only knows. But I remember the feeling of immense satisfaction when, armed with all four hot properties under my arm, I crept back home in smuggler mode.

My bedroom was the scene of a crime of the stomach. Over the next few hours, I repeatedly went back upstairs to eat 'just one last one' from the array of goodies behind the clothes in the back of my wardrobe. Narnia had nothing on me. By bedtime they were gone. The last few were forcibly eaten by telling myself that it would be best to finish the rest now, because then no one would know, no evidence at the scene of the crime. And after all – guess what - tomorrow I would be back on the diet - the one that would work this time.

I'd even have countless bad dreams about getting this unbearable panic in the pit of my stomach because I feared I wouldn't get my share of the food, doubtless linked to finding empty cake packets once too often in the kitchen because my brothers and sister got there before me.

Tip - in a family of six or seven, packets of five cakes isn't too clever.

Oh the countless bad dreams about not getting in the queue quickly enough, or being in the wrong queue, or not being able to get to the rest of the food before it was cleared away, etc etc etc. Never once do I recall feeling genuinely happy around food, or fulfilled. The shame of it is that it was all learned behavior. 'Cos – would it really have mattered?

Did my body truly want to overeat? No, it was all in my mind. What's the worst that could happen if I missed out on my share? I'd have to eat something else. Or be hungry for a little longer. God forbid we should feel hungry.

Chapter Eight - Hunger Know Thyself

Two more keys to help you escape from food prison!

- Treat hunger as a friend.

- Don't practise prevention eating.

In Food Prison, we're terrified of hunger. We fear it as if it would strike us down should we let its probing claws gnaw away at our stomachs for more than a couple of seconds, We panic. We stuff food in our mouths and once we've started, we just keep doing it. So to avoid it, we take precautions - it's called prevention eating, "in case I don't get the chance to eat later on."

Hunger is one of the body's most basic signals that it's time for fuel. You need to feel it, and you shouldn't eat before you do. So don't eat before you are properly hungry, and don't carry on eating after you're *satisfied.* Hunger shouts, remember, so you will definitely know you're hungry. Other signs apart from distinct pangs include:

- Feeling slightly giddy.

- Feeling a little sick.

- Feeling a little panicky.

- Feeling that you can't concentrate.

There are medical reasons for each of these alternative signs of being hungry, and all you need to do is experiment a little. Wait. Observe. Note it for next time. Play the scientist. Conduct your own observational tests to see which sign means what for you. Think, "what's my body trying to tell me here?"

This is a biggie - it could just be, "I'm thirsty." If we are, it's possibly the reason for many of the signals our body gives out during the day, since many of us are so dehydrated the chemical and electrical reactions in our bodies just can't work properly. So they send out distress signals, which manifest themselves as a multitude of different symptoms. Including hunger.

Best treatment? If you're not distinctly hungry, but something isn't quite right and you feel you need to take some action? Drink a big glass of water. Sounds simplistic, but you'll soon know if it was hunger, because it'll be back again in fifteen minutes or so. At which point you could eat some food, but listen to your body's next signal and only choose what it's really crying out for - what your body wants, not what your mind thinks your body wants. Imagine the food in your mouth. Smell it. Even taste a tiny bit if needs be. Imagine it in your stomach having eaten it. Does it feel right? Then try it. Don't do anything else at the same time, just sit and savour every mouthful. Don't get the next one ready till you've swallowed the first. Give your body a chance to start reacting to the food being eaten rather than wolfing it down before your body's even noticed it's coming, Then you're more likely to notice 'satisfied'. Eating was designed to be pleasurable, like sex, also necessary for the survival of the species, so it's no accident these vital 'tasks' feel so good! Then monitor what's happening to your body and stop when the taste of the food suddenly isn't 'blow your mind fantastic' anymore. It can still taste good, but not incredible, so stop. Yes, I said stop! Especially when you start noticing your own most distinctive signs.

You may take a deep breath. You may start being distracted by what's going on around you. When you haven't yet eaten enough, eating will be the only thing on your mind, believe me. When your mind starts wandering off onto other topics, you're probably satisfied. You'll have waited, of course, till you were hungry in the first place, and the rewards of the resulting heightened pleasure for the taste buds, near ecstasy sometimes, will be yours for the taking. Food Freedom brings with it the most wonderful eating experiences. You're not feeling deprived, possibly for the first time in your adult life. You're choosing what your body wants most each and every time. What tastes best, each and every time. You can, if you choose (that is if it's what your body wants) have anything because nothing is forbidden. You're not eating things just for the sake of it, or because you feel you have to, or because it's still sitting there looking at you, or because you've always reached out automatically and said ‘yes’ without thinking, because you've been so used to saying ‘yes’ if it meant allowing yourself a little unexpected treat. Emotional eating will be no more. This is a biggie as I was to find out in later months. Forbidden territory will be no more, and you are having the unique experience, almost certainly for the first time you can remember, of stopping eating when you still feel comfortable. **Stop when you're satisfied.**

Maybe even leave a little on your plate. Yippee it's possible! That's Food Freedom in a nutshell, and if you want to try it out, then start right away. See if you can do it at the next mealtime. Take a few baby steps towards a giant leap of faith that will set you free of food prison forever. And you can start by waiting till you're really hungry the next time you eat. See the later guidelines, some specifically for people who choose at this stage to combine it with existing diet plans, and get stuck in. And keep listening back to the tapes again and again, to reinforce the new behaviour.(6) **You'll never change a lifetime's bad habits by listening just once.**

-It's deciding to do it.

- Taking action to make it happen.

- Then reinforcing that new behaviour again and again.

- Then relying on the Support System Treats to help you find other coping mechanisms and to make the changes permanent.

Just remember that those closest to you may find it all a little perplexing.

Chapter Nine - What 'They' Say

Even your children can break free from the pattern if you do it first.

More slings and arrows, I'm afraid.

You might change you, but you won't change them as readily, especially not overnight, unless they're really open-minded, or desperate to change! So just accept that some people in your life will just have to learn later than others, and only tell them in detail when you feel the time is right, when they start asking about your new outlook, or your new shape. So many people live their lives based on other people's opinions. I did as well to be honest. Others' opinions were the most important thing in my decision making process. So if I heard too loud and too clear that others thought I was wrong, I'd just give up. Why do you think we took on board all these erroneous rules about eating in the first place? We must have believed their perpetrators to be right, or we would have ignored their comments and 'advice'. But thing is, a lot of our habits stem from having our beliefs overruled from a young age.

I can never say all this enough. Think about it.

- *"Don't trust your body to get it right, trust me."*

- *"Mummy knows best."*

- *"Why do you want to eat that now, put it back."*

- *"You're in my house and you will do as I say."*

- *"Why? Because I said so. "Oh dear, oh dear, oh dear."*

Don't feel too bad if you recognise yourself in any of this, I was a 'worst offender' because I was just doing what my mum and peers and siblings had done to me. And so the cycle continues.

Unless you break the cycle by becoming aware right now.

It'll be the best gift you could ever give someone, especially a child. To not have them 'unlearn' their body's perfect eating signals. Wow, what a thought. Do you recall any memories of weird behaviour around food? Linked to deprivation and control? Why would a new human being, born with a perfect eating mechanism completely override their body and its signals, to participate in such bizarre food rituals? Why do we do it to ourselves? Why do we do it to our children? My mum, bless her, is a chief offender. She does it as a matter of course, quite naturally, when confronted with the enemy - food. And just like many chief offenders, she vehemently denies it. I recall once commenting to her about a book we'd interviewed someone about on Live at Three with Jayne Irving on Living in 1997. It was basically saying that you're the results of your mum's eating habits - if she dieted, then you as her daughter will almost certainly repeat the sins of the mother in your adult life. It makes sense. You see it happen, assume that's how things are done, and fall naturally into that pattern when your time comes. Say the same things, make the same observations, feel the same guilt, lose a few pounds, gain a lot, lose a few, gain a lot, and end up looking just like her eventually. Words of wisdom from a mother's lips are taken as gospel, especially when you're too young to know better, subconsciously shaping our ritual beliefs and determining our food destiny.

So I told mum about this book and its claim. "I haven't got a food problem." she indignantly replied, "I could tell you everything I've eaten for the last two days." That's my mum, indignant, "I know what to do, I know what I should and shouldn't eat," she declares, merrily delving into my fridge as soon as she walks in through the door. Mostly cuddly or voluptuous through the years, and sometimes really big and buxom, my lovely old dad loved every bit of her, 'his bit of meat.' But at her largest she seemed very unhappy. She'd eaten her way there through five children and a complete lack of understanding of portion sizes, and now fashion dictated she should be slim. So she basically joined the yo-yo brigade from there on in. She did get really thin one year. She and my sister did - with Weight Watchers. Oh if only we could wave wands overnight - wouldn't things be different? I bet she wished she'd stayed there at that skinny weight, looking slightly emaciated with no bust to speak of, but fitting into skinnies' clothes and feeling good when she looked in the mirror, and feeling crap when she looked in the fridge. Vikki Hansen was a slimming club instructor and has grave doubts about the long-term losses sustained by club members. According to findings, over 90% of the people put it right back on again. So they really are still food prisoners when they have lost the weight, left the class and gone back to being 'normal'.(7) So many of us know people like that. Or we are people like that.

Isn't it true? The phrase, "I really must go back to slimming club," in one form or another, has been heard time and time again through the years. The same people. The same problem back again, the same ten or twenty pounds to lose.

Break the pattern. Break out of that food prison.

Get Food Freedom and you will stay out, permanently. It's so easy. Really. So many people can testify to how permanent this system is. And do you know why? Why it's so logical and it works? Because it's eating the way nature intended. Eating the way you were born to. Kids, young kids, left to choose their own food from a selection, chose a balanced diet over the course of the week. After the first few days of eating all the junk - and that's only because they've already been subject to some form of deprivation and control - they then actually chose to eat the veggies as well as the meat, the fruit as well as the pies, and sometimes they only ate the fruit, or the salad, or the broccoli. Dare you try it with your own kids? I tell you what, it's really liberating, to not have to stand guard at the door of their stomachs and to not have to chastise or goad or bribe or threaten your way through mealtimes. Give it a go, and you'll set them on the path to freedom for the rest of their lives too. If you still don't see the value of this to yourself, if, for instance, you've been trying it for a few weeks and haven't quite got the hang of 'satisfied' yet, don't give up, your family need you to stop your vicious food cycle, they need you to be happy, don't they? You owe it to them, and yourself, to keep trying. So if this is your second or third listening, just persevere.

And, stop beating yourself up about it all. Relax. Get calm. See it through. Work out what's been missing, adjust, and step right on up to the next level. The pace of change is completely individual. Some people can notice big differences quite quickly whereas others sometimes put on a little before it starts to come off, gradually getting the hang of the eating the Freedom way, and becoming a totally different person around food.

Examples

Another example comes in the form of my own experiences with slimming clubs. As someone who hates being told what to do, it makes me want to do it more. The very thought of going to a club I'm not looking forward to anyway, where there's a chance someone could be telling me I've been 'bad' this last week, and scrawling in a little unhappy face into my record book, then sitting talking about the very thing we're trying to make less important in our lives in order to become 'normal' - food - and what we are allowed, and what foods are ‘sins'. Well, God knows why I even bothered going to that very first club back in the Dark Days of Screensport in Cheshire. Desperation I suppose. I'd got to the stage where I was eating food from the bin, that spag bol I described earlier on. I'd gone to get slimming pills. I'd come off the pill to lose that quarter of a stone it had put on me a couple of years earlier. I'd done the gym thing. I'd tried the f-plan (and we all know what happened with that one!) And nothing worked. This was also the time that mum and Linda my sister had done so well. They were skinny, I was really, really heavy, and self-conscious about it too, and they nagged me.

"It's worked for us," they cried, unable to see why their way was not going to work for me. Linda had just become a club instructor herself, her great big fat picture from a few years earlier sat in my bedroom looking at me every time I came back for a visit to mum's. So off I went. It was a local club in Northwich, and pleasing to my eye when I walked in the door and saw loads and loads of people far fatter than me. But they were the ones smiling when in week three, I'd actually gained back the two pounds I'd lost the week before, plus an extra one into the bargain. Must have been someone else's is all I can say! And the chat wasn't great either, just obvious stuff I really did know. And there lies the problem. There must be few serial dieters who don't know most of what we should do. The problem is getting yourself to do it consistently. As Anthony Robbins says, keep saying, "I should do this, I should do that," and pretty soon you'll have 'should' all over yourself.(9) 'I should' belongs on 'I'll try' street. You can make the decision in an instant, for instance to give up smoking. It's the sticking to it afterwards that can be the problem. The 'challenge', should we say.

And that's where Food Freedom really comes into its own.

Because what you're looking at is adopting a whole new thought process, a whole new way of eating, a whole new permanent system to help you break free and get liberated. And stay there. Once you start doing it, the weight coming off is the side effect of adopting a new, healthy approach to food and mealtimes, rather than the primary aim. What you end up doing is actually the very thing you'd started overriding all those years ago.

That's why this system is so different from any other.

My research into what's around included a couple of tape sets from the States. Very intense they were, too. They had a few things in common with some of the ones I researched from the UK, mainly the visualisation techniques and affirmations, and I believe there's a lot to be said for all that. After all, it's definitely true that what you focus on expands, so if you say you're going to lose weight, but inside you actually believe you're a fat person, you'll almost certainly break the diet at the first hurdle. It's going to take a lot of mind-conditioning to shake free the deep down opinion that you're useless, you 'always' eat too much, you 'never' lose weight no matter what you do. But it's possible. Unless you have a medical condition, the only way you stay fat is by eating more than you use up in energy on a consistent basis. The only way you will lose weight is by eating less than you have been, as well as preferably, exercising more, and now Food Freedom to keep it off for good. But a traditional diet of deprivation and control leads to a lowered metabolism as your body trips into famine mode, Yo-yo dieting through the years will never work long-term, and will lead to stress galore.

Forget the diets forever if you learn Food Freedom, and gradually go back to trusting your body to guide you in choosing what, when and how much to eat. But how did we get here in the first place? Was your life like mine?

Chapter Ten - More From the Fat Lady

The biography continued - Bridget Jones eat your heart out.

I'll never forget my first encounters with Freedom Eating. The turnaround happened in the Spring of 1999. A couple of Eureka moments tied in with the arrival of the ladies from America and an insight I'll never forget. My job at QVC the Shopping Channel source of stress and so much of the weight gain over the past five years - was now the source of my salvation. The two guests Shawn Goodman and Vikki Hansen, appeared on air with their book and tape pack, telling us all about the way they now lived their lives without worrying about weight gain, or food, or calories. The system was called Freedom Eating.

Ha ha ha, funny joke - you're free to eat what you want, that's right, isn't it? That's what everyone says, and it's true. But the crucial difference here is the 'want' bit. I read the book with interest. 'The Seven Secrets of Slim People ... ' hmmm. **Eat till you're satisfied, not till you're full.** I did the show immediately after their first appearance, and spoke about this on air. "What," said Mrs thirteen stone, "you mean you don't keep eating till you can't breathe anymore?" Ha ha, funny fat lady. Again.

But the book had me hooked, and I really and truly started to see a way out of the eternal food prison in which I'd made my permanent HQ and set up camp. That summer, until their next visit, and my first show with them, I semi-practiced it. You know you always think it's your little secret - people don't realise how bad this food thing really is for you. You have to deal with it alone, or in secret, or you're a failure. Well, surprise, surprise, you're not alone. You're just like me, and if I can do it, you can do it, and I am doing it. After twenty long years of 'having a food problem', I'm at last finding out the secrets of slim people. And the good news is - we can be like them. Keep a diary, like I did, to chart your progress.

At the time of writing this section, I'm nine and a half pounds lighter. It all actually seems to be working - you really can have the best of both worlds -be 'normal' around food and eat what you like, and have a great shape! Well, I'm moving in the right direction. Two inches off my waist so far: it's doing my morale, and my sex life, the world of good. I'm starting to see my ribs again. The weight loss equivalent in pounds of lard which I keep as a visual reminder of what I've lost, is growing and growing, only now I'm carrying it in a bag and not on me, and the insights I've been collecting over the last six months have been and continue to be illuminating. The first insight was around the time I first saw the girls and their system on QVC. At home, we'd had marriage problems, and come through them.

And at the heart of my problem was the reasoning, "If only I was slim then he'd want me more and there wouldn't be a problem. If I was able to eat normally then everything would be ok." Familiar one, huh? Well, me and The Man were in the kitchen and I was, as usual, sounding off about weight and food and blah blah blah. And he chirps up: "But you eat quite normally, don't you. It's not like you're always eating rubbish, you eat quite healthily really, don't you?" Stunned silence. Me and the 'N' word in the same sentence, in the same sentence as eating habits. I thought about it long and hard. Well, actually, yes, I did usually eat healthily. I didn't stuff myself every night. You know the amazing before and after pictures in the paper about slimmers of the year who have shed ten stone and they got there in the first place by gorging on chips and curries and beer and chocolate. That was never me. But I thought of myself in the same terms as they did, no doubt.

- "Jerry Springer, I have a food problem."

- "I see. Well, pardon me for saying it, but Debbie, you don't even look fat."

- "But I am fat, Jerry. I've been bad."

- "Well, see how you feel when we bring on Angela. Angela - come on out here. You see, Angela's over twenty stone - 280lb - ***now*** *look at her and say* ***you've*** *got a problem ... a problem, a problem."*

Like a dream sequence, it all unfolds in my mind. How can I possibly class myself as having a problem, when I'm nowhere near as bad as others, Can't explain that one. So what do we do? We just put up, shut up, and eat up, always in solitude, always in guilt city, but invariably with supreme satisfaction when the food is in our mouths and going down bit by precious bit.

This technique set me free. Full stop. Period. End of story. You just have to follow the guidelines, and find some faith in your own body that it knows what to choose, and how much to opt for, without ever again needing to reprimand or lecture yourself, or class whole categories of food as off bounds. It's working so far. But it's still early days, and there's actually no reason to think that your gradual weight loss will stop as long as you're listening to your body and eating the way nature intended, until your body reaches its ideal weight. Its own natural weight, which may not be the weight which you'd like, but this way at least you break free from food prison for the rest of your life. Because I've changed my eating habits - easy bit. But I'm sticking to it - hard bit, but I'm not on a diet, or counting, or beating myself up- good bit. I'm getting guidance from a proven, reliable source - easy bit, but I'm putting it into action - challenging bit. I know what I should do. Knowing's the easy bit, right? And it always has been, it's doing it that's the problem. But this time I'm not having the eternal torture of sabotaging myself at the slightest provocation, you know the form - I've eaten one biscuit too many so I'll blow the diet, eat the lot and start again tomorrow. How many 'last suppers' have you had in your time? I'm calmer, more full of conviction that I know this time is different, this time I'll do it. Instead of beating myself up about it every time I stray off the track or make the slightest mistake. I'm happy going through the process of changing my life. And boy is there a lot of change in store. Changing the habits of a lifetime.

In 1974, the girls in 2H who brought an apple in for break time didn't mind giving me their cores when they'd had enough after only eating half. The school dinners were bliss and heaven: caramel tart, manchester tart, the best custard on the planet, never yet equalled, subject of many a hard-done-by / don't get in in time for the sitting and severe angst from not getting my share type dream. Morden Farm Middle School in south London had a canteen second to none and it had a lot to answer for!

I wouldn't mind, but I wasn't actually fat. In fact, I was one of the slimmer ones in the family for a long time. I remember Dad giving me jip one night over how far my collar bones were protruding, and I recall feeling proud that for once in my life someone was using the 's' word on me! Skinny? No way! Only the stick insects in the class, who looked like their legs would break if you so much as looked at them on the hockey pitch, were usually associated with the S word. Oh how I dreamed of being skinny.

When I was nine I drew pictures of myself, imagining what I'd be like at age thirteen, how I thought I'd have changed by then: skinny, with boobs and a boyfriend called Michael (for some reason). None of which turned out to be true. I ended up four years later, a slightly taller version of how I was at nine. With a little bit more podge round the middle consisting solely of marmalade on toast by then. And the boyfriend was called Neil Develin. Then Robert D, then Robert E, then Rob Squires. Maybe boys called Robert were attracted to chubby kids with a penchant for marmalade, I don't know.

Why is it that all my memories of school trips seem to be punctuated with meal times? The delicious confiture, croissants, and cafe-au-lait from Dravail, just outside Paris, where we all went aged eleven or twelve. The spaghetti and first Martini and lemonade ever, in Andalo, whilst skiing at age fourteen. The theatre trip with the girls up town to see Tom Conti in, *Whose Life is it Anyway*, at sixteen, which couldn't take place until I'd stopped the taxi to buy up the sweet shop. And of course, the *piece de resistance*, close encounters of the Pontins kind, the holiday camp never knew what hit it the year they brought in self-service and my family arrived and served themselves to some of every option on the menu - every mealtime, When we got home we were all half a stone heavier, to be expected on holiday though, wasn't it?

There were countless other memories too, of course. But why did we have the obsession with food? Well the obvious reply is being in a big family. I was the eldest of five, after all. Remember, Mum and Dad went shopping on a Friday. By Monday, all the best stuff was gone – guaranteed. This was the thing, if you didn't eat it there and then, irrespective of whether you were hungry or not, you would miss out. And we all became very skilled at overriding our appetites and our body's signals, to allow our brain to take charge. Eat it now or you go without. Let's make a move body, or we might not get a second chance. And our body said "ok."

-"Here, have another packet of crisps - there are only two packs left." And our body said "ok."

-"I say, body, there are two more courses after this, are you sure you don't mind me getting another piece of garlic bread with your appetiser?"

And our body said, "I don't know, you tell me, brain you're the boss."

And so it happens that we all *stop* listening to our bodies and do what we think instead of pausing for a minute and considering doing what our bodies *feel* like. Listening to our own needs. God forbid we should ever take any notice of our body's suggestions that we don't really want any more food just yet. Don't be so stupid, just open your mouth and *eat*.

But the worst times were still to come. Still really finding my feet in the fatty stakes and on the whole not doing too badly at fifteen, I'd got down to an all-time low of nine stone following an apple a day diet, at lunchtime, and a child size portion of dinner at night. Or an egg and a fish finger for lunch, taken to school in a Tupperware container. In bed by 9pm, stomach growling, Or cursing myself if I'd succumbed to temptation and committed the heinous crime of giving in to a bowl of - shock, horror - cornflakes. Every carefully-counted calorie imprinted on my memory, or recorded in my five year diary, Bridget Jones style. So I did, in fact, briefly manage to achieve a really flat stomach, and for a few short months, felt like I was truly one of the Slim People. In the mirror I was, but in the brain I was still the troubled fattie who could never be normal around food. I was fifteen, and being slim lasted two years.

At fourteen, I'd been in with a bunch of girls who all had similar hang-ups. I'd pigged out that summer, and had a horrendous photo taken of me with the rest of the mostly slim and nubile borough hockey team on our tour to Holland. I even remember sneaking downstairs in the middle of the night to pinch a few Quality Street from a big tin kept by our unsuspecting host family. No one ever knew but me. And boy was I thrilled at my booty, three toffees and my favourite purple wrapped caramel one with the nut in the middle. If only they knew. Apeldoorn never knew what hit it when I returned the following year a stone lighter, a tornado on the hockey pitch, and raring to get off with whomever I could in the boys team, off the pitch. A subsequent memory involved kissing each of the boys in turn on the coach on the way home and feeling terribly guilty when Dad found out. Guilt in those days equalled several packets of Rancheros crisps and two Twixes, I seem to remember.

Anyway, still pretty trim due to all the sport, and however diet obsessed, by seventeen, I was now celebrating every birthday or anniversary, or family business getting its first bank loan, with a meal out. Mostly with my first long-term, official, grown-up working boyfriend Martin, and mostly at *The Safari Steak House* in Morden.

So here we were, I remember it so well. Prawn cocktail, then fillet steak, buttery jacket potato, peas and onion rings. Bread and butter. Diet bitter lemon (got to make some effort, huh), and their speciality dessert, the gut-busting banana split, to follow. Coffee with lots of cream and sugar, mints, and on this occasion even a little cheese and biscuits, and a sick bag. I was never one for a drink, but Martin polished off a couple of lagers on top of all that, but then he'd actually left some of his other courses, some of which was also polished off by me. We stood. We paid. We walked out into the night air and then it hit me. I was so stuffed I had to walk up and down a bit outside before I could actually bend enough, without being sick, to get in the car for the journey home. At least ten minutes of the walking before I could trust myself to face the five minute car journey back to my house without turning into a scene out of the movie *Car Wash*.

So there was the pattern. Reinforcement that this was the way things should be and every flaming time an occasion arose, my brain took over my body like a woman possessed. "The famine has ended! The famine has ended!" went the cry, and the body metaphorically ran around like the proverbial blue-bummed fly, acting accordingly. I probably ate enough calories on those occasions, to last me three days. Then go back to being 'normal' or 'good' which equated to being on a diet, or 'bad' which equated to not following a diet.

In fact, I was eating normally, but not realising it, and punishing myself in the extreme if I strayed from the strict rules I'd laid down for my eating patterns. Severe Rules which are another big no-no for successful weight loss. You must have suspected by now that the key to Food Freedom is to unlearn all the bad things, all the unnatural things, which you've learned about food through the years.

Control and deprivation don't work - long term.

Endless charts of unrealistic weight losses went on the wall. And soon got taken off again when there was no more room to keep changing all the dates on it, as each successive deadline came and went to no avail. One of the only other times after my school years I ever really got slim was when I was on Larry Grayson's Easter Generation Game on TV in 1981. I reached a lovely 9st 13lb, but was totally one hundred per cent screwed up about it. "Does my bum look big in this?" wasn't the half of it. Said boyfriend Martin endured endless paranoia and demands for comparisons with other girls' body parts. He was having to contend with an undergraduate trainee accountant who spent all day bored silly and looking forward to a lunchtime Caramac chocolate bar, eaten slowly and savoured religiously. Interspersed with frenzied bouts of bookkeeping to make up for the lost time I'd spent daydreaming about the rosy future I was creating for myself, and dreams of TV beckoned. So did another boyfriend, eventually. Mark had a penchant for muesli and also scrambled eggs on doorstep toast, and a mum who made amazing cakes. But I was working my way through university at the time by cleaning loos and keeping Sainsbury's spic and span for Dad's new contract cleaning business.

All that work helped keep the weight off, to an extent, but all that extra physical work gave me a new license to consume.

If only I'd have learned then what I know now. If only someone had sat me down and explained what I found out when I discovered Food Freedom. The logic. The liberation. The lunches. By the summer of 1983, I'd scraped through University (too many distractions in the form of theatre, an attempt at modelling, singing, and boyfriends), and managed to fit into two small suits bought for all those job interviews I was going to get once I left the London School of Economics, but none came. Too late I realised I wasn't going to get any of the high-flying positions I wanted in advertising or at the BBC or as a producer, without having been the Head Journalist on the London Student Magazine, or creator of an award winning university drama transferred to the Edinburgh Festival, or top student 1983. I'd only managed to reach co-features editor and to play Hortense in the LSE production of The Boyfriend which someone else had produced. And even then my legs were too fat. Why were all the other girls' legs always so much slimmer? Now I look back and wish I could wave a wand and have stayed the shape I was then. If only the control and deprivation hadn't set in in the next few years and taken my weight swings to an even greater level.

Before I left University, I managed to diet and Slendertone my way into a couple of Miss Pontins finals competitions, and was quite proud of the fact I'd got there, even though standing next to the others, I knew I had no chance. Scored a couple of Twix and Rolo sessions for that one, I can tell you! But there were still no job interviews, and a life of cross casting and balance sheets spread out before me, unless I did something. And Mark was on the way out by then too, so I had to get my act together. So I sold my motorbike and paid for a three month 'How to be a radio presenter' course at the National Broadcasting School in Soho, London. Still living at home, I totally immersed myself in this new world. I had lots of barriers to overcome, but not a spare second to even consider comfort-eating.

Before too long I was doing all the hours that God sends, practising after-hours in their studios, surviving on the odd yoghurt and packet of chips from the kebab shop on the comer of Greek Street, or once in a blue moon, a Topic bar. Every night I'd come home late, exhilarated, exhausted, and excited about the next day's experiences, my head in the clouds dreaming of becoming a 'proper' presenter with a 'proper' job. Oh, and of a fellow student called Andy. The weight fell off - I was busy and happy.

By Christmas, we were all unleashed onto the unsuspecting radio community (only two or three getting or already having jobs) the rest of us going back to what we'd done before, all the while perfecting our radio showreels and sending off applications all over the country. Rejection time. Despite my winning their Student with Most Progress Award, rejection time - big time. Oh, and Andy didn't love me. I forgave him years later when it turned out he was gay - but that didn't help me at the time, but, euphoria - it was Christmas! The time of year when food abounds, just asking to be eaten to excess, the perfect antidote to all that rejection. That Christmas, the weight piled on, and I went blonde. By the January, at a reunion evening out, one of my fellow students didn't recognise me from behind. So sad. I went blonder, tried to get some dress sense, went back to the accountants, and spent the next five months tearing my heart out over Andy, who saw me regularly but at arms length... most of the time. I wrote reams and reams of soul-searching, heart-string- pulling prose for him, none of which worked, apart from to make me feel better temporarily by getting it all out, and to set up a pattern that was to repeat itself on a regular basis for the next fifteen years of my life. I added things up by machine, in neat columns all day, dreamed of Andy all night, and ate chocolate, biscuits and pizzas to lighten the load. And put on nearly a stone.

Then I discovered diet pills. By May 1984, I was winging my way to Corfu for my first ever foreign holiday with my (slim) mate Gill and her (slim) sister and her sister's (skinny) friend. By late May 1984, I was winging my way back again, half a stone heavier (a neat achievement in two weeks considering my determination not to), and about to start a whole new era for myself working for a fledgling sports cable TV company called Screensport in Knutsford, Cheshire. The big move, leaving home at last.

Auntie Peggy offered me a room for a couple of months, and I gratefully took up her offer, finding, to my delight, that I was able to successfully challenge myself to eat all her goodies, and more, including the new found delight of northern bakeries and vanilla slices. Just how much weight could I put on? Eleven and a half stone was easy. Nudging eleven and three quarters, bulimia finally came knocking on my door. Soon after, and left to my own devices, in the solitude of my own house in Wincham near Northwich and two and a half hours from home, looking after myself was super stressful - my very first household bills! Eek! Still no boyfriend except Andy, sort of, and long distance, and trying to have the so-called great single life. This was the worst time for my loss of control.

Don't get me wrong - as any high achiever in a similar situation knows - you can channel your energies as well as the next person so that everyone thinks you're successful and happy. And you probably are - to a certain extent. But when food's got a grip, logic goes out the window. Especially at the end of the day behind closed doors, when the only person you've got to impress is yourself, and you've never understood that bit of life at all.

What is it that makes a self-respecting adult become so controlled by the need to eat that they crave food they can't have, don't stock it so they can't binge on it, but then cave in and leave the house late at night to drive round and round in search of a Topic or a Chippy? What is it that makes them choose a best friend who's skinny (albeit as neurotic as I was but for different reasons)? But the difference in size between me and my mate Jax didn't exactly help me solve the boyfriend dilemma when we went clubbing together. Or on a Scottish skiing holiday where the really attractive ski instructor asked her to dance at the final night do and not me. Not me, the thirteen stone fuchsia pink ski-suited Mrs Blobby hurtling down the ski slopes in a permanent snow plough. Can't understand why he chose her not me. I didn't really go back and stuff my face silly that night, did I? Lying in bed listening to '99 Red Balloons', or Go West, or Alison Moyet's 'Ole Devil Called Love, with my packets of shortbread and bags of crisps, I knew I'd hit rock bottom.

I'd hit an all-time high of over thirteen stone by the time I came back and had started to feel the rolls of fat on my back, not just round my waist, but up around my shoulders, weird thing that was. In later years, I'd hit it again, although the next time I was carrying a ten pound baby, at the time, however, I was finally despondent.

Chapter Eleven - Emotional Eating

The reasons I eventually ballooned.

The dinner party with the infamous bin-scavenging episode happened that spring, I think. Friends from Screensport came to my house and were treated to Spag Bol a la Debbie. They came, they ate, they left some, they went home again. I cleared up, confidently binning the leftovers and leaving the washing up till morning.

So why couldn't I just go to sleep? I'd managed to get as far as chucking the goddam food away - wasn't that enough? Why couldn't those next few hours have passed with a satiated appetite, both for food (I'd naturally had over large portions myself anyway) and for company? And why was I drawn like a magnet to those ample leftovers from skinny people, solidifying into a mass of cold stodge languishing in the bin and calling me from my dreams.

- *"You know we're here!"*

- *"You know your number one rule is never to waste food."*

- *"You think there'll be a famine tomorrow, you think you have to finish everything off - even other people's leftovers, like there's a war on. Just like when you were at home - the family always cleaned their plates. You were 'good' children for eating it all then. You were told you had to eat it all."*

- *"Yeah, so stop kidding yourself, and give in and come and get us out of this bin - now."*

After all, it would just be this once, then you'd never do it again, right? I'd have been a fully-fledged bulimic but I could never bring myself to throw it up again and waste it. I think the only time I stooped lower than that was when I was determined not to go out in search of food. So I ate everything I could get my hands on within the house, including some old defrosted bits of leftover pastry I'd put in the freezer rather than bear to throw it away. Another error; you can waste it and throw it away rather than force your body to eat it if you've had enough. But maybe it was because I'd had an insight into the depths to which I'd plummet that night. Microwaved, soggy and pasty ... mmm ...

feast fit for a king - well for a sad cow in need of some serious help, anyway. And why did this happen so frequently - so much that eventually it became part of the fabric of every day of my life? The answer was obvious, it was emotional eating - comfort eating. I lived alone, I wasn't in a relationship, so I simply fed my pangs of loneliness and angst with food - using all the learned behaviours I'd been studying for so long.

Soon after, my fortunes changed slightly with a brand new job, and it started to feel like the old days at broadcasting school as I threw myself into the job as broadcast assistant at Piccadilly Radio in Manchester. I was in seventh heaven. The first eight months were a dream time. At last I was in broadcasting and headed in the right direction. Whether as one of Timmy Mallett's helpers (where Chris Evans also began), or vetting Steve Penk's early wind-up callers, I loved every minute of it. Hardly thought about my weight. It was far easier to subsist on ready-meals and fruit. I finally landed an overnight show of my own and a future husband from the sales department called Tony. Tall, dark, handsome, no food problem in sight, he and I hit it off over a badminton court and the rest, as they say is 'His' Story. My story was always fleshed out in private as I fought to deal with my eating problems to a greater or lesser degree.

Hunger for companionship satisfied, I gradually worked my way out of the eating disorders borne of loneliness and stress and pressure on myself to achieve, and by the time we moved back down to London for my new wonder job as Phillip Schofield's replacement and the first female in the broom cupboard on Children's BBC, I was regaining some semblance of normality. What are you hungry for, really, when you eat? Is it really the food, or is it something else?

For the next seven years, I kept my weight down to a healthy ten and a half stone - slim for me and give or take a couple of pounds, the odd post-holiday blowout or a Christmas or a pregnancy, I stayed there. Life was good, albeit Tone and I took it in turns to work, more or less: it always seemed he or I would lose a job or be made redundant in turn. We rarely got to sustain the income, never paid off debts, except with new loans. But we were fine, on the whole. And the kids were great. Although this book might not mention it as much, I tend towards being a happy, contented little soul, and we were doing fine as our little family unit established itself as three, then four, and domestic routine was a welcome break from the pressure to achieve, and part of what became my day to day life.

In September 1990, Lauren was now one year old and I'd got back down to about 10st 5lbs. Felt great, looked fine, did a Dr. Who weekend on my current fab job on what was BSB (remember the squarials)? So I can't blame the pregnancies. I could lay a few shovelfuls of blame at the door of comfort eating as a result of Rupert Murdoch's takeover of BSB though. We all got made redundant in the November. Tony and I felt like we were back to square one. I don't think what happened as a consequence of that really ever allowed us to recover from it - we've been up and down ever since, really, and so has my helter skelter of weight loss and gain - till now.

There were some definite highlights, however. I auditioned for a new show called Stars in Their Eyes as Sheena Easton - they said "lose some weight." I did but not enough, and although I sounded like Sheena Easton, I still looked like Eartha Kitt but it was great fun to take part in. My weight was then a low, low 10 stone 2lb, temporarily through diet pills, diuretic tablets and crash diets, but that was the last time I got to that weight, and, as ever, it was short-lived.

Now I'd like to be that weight again, but the reality is, my body might not want to be. If my natural weight is a slightly rounded 10 and a half stone, then that's what I'll tend towards, however much I fight it. Another reality check for the terminally hungry. So along the way there were highs and lows, ups and downs, good times and not so good. Dad dying was a bit of a bummer - another story for another time. But basically it was cancer of the liver in 1992, six months and he was gone. Just like that. It's ok now, I can and I like to talk about him fondly, but as everyone knows who's going through bereavement, there aren't any easy answers.

Two years later I landed the job at QVC the newly launched Shopping Channel in Battersea, London. Great for cash-flow, bad for life balance, zen and me-time. Within another two years I was back up to over eleven stone. By 1998, I'd reached twelve and a half, and so as not to break the pattern, by Spring of 1999 I was nearer thirteen, maybe even thirteen and a half. I'd stopped getting on the scales by then. I thought it can't be long before I got to my pre-birth pregnancy weight. The only difference being I wasn't carrying a 10lb 9oz baby. All I needed was a fuchsia pink ski suit and history would have come full circle.

Now a lot of other things happened alongside this continual weight problem, culminating in a near-miss marriage break up in early 1999. But again, that's another story. Suffice it to say my friends and relations helped me pull through and got me and Tony back on the straight and narrow. And that's maybe what became the catalyst for knowing I had to shake free from the noose of food prison. When having a food problem is pulling you down, you can't think or act straight. When food prison's your home, natural body functions can be over-ridden like a shot, at the prospect of a slap up meal, or a bit of short-lived comfort. Especially when you're not getting what you need elsewhere, in terms of affection, attention or excitement in your life. I'm sure you've all got your own versions.

If your hunger is not really for food, you satiate your needs the only way you know how. The old familiar way that's been with you much of your life - through food. That fleeting pleasure is tangible, if only for a few minutes each time. It's physical. It's controlled by you, it's your decision to go and eat the next thing, and the next, and the next. Because every time is the last time, right? As the experts say when so much in your life is out of your control, no wonder you feel the need to be the one putting yourself consciously in the driving seat at meal time, and any time in between.

In a natural state, our bodies would signal that it's time for us to eat by giving us hunger pangs. Then we'd eat a little, enough for the hunger pangs to stop, till the food tasting so unbelievably good definitely subsides, till we feel comfortable but not so we can feel the food-in our belly. Definitely not till we can't breathe anymore. We'd eat till we're satisfied. Satisfied. Not full. Not bursting. Then we'd go off and do whatever else we needed to do without another thought about the food. Ideally, food wouldn't be that important - till the next meal time. But when everything that controls that process is completely imbalanced, when you're used to overriding your body's signals and you tell it when to eat, not the other way round, making it eat when it's not ready for food - like the petrol tank that's not empty yet - the overflow has to go somewhere, and it's usually deposited as fat on the body. How the hell can you have food problems and hope never to have weight trouble? Million dollar question - and don't believe anyone who says they have it all sussed.

So by May 1999, I was ready to change.

They say when the student is ready the teacher will appear. Never more for me than this last year (commencing in the spring of 1999). Some of the best advice I've ever heard has all come along this year. Mostly on various audio tapes. I'll list at the back some of the books and tapes I'd recommend, which have most impressed me and impacted in some way on my life. Not just the ones about weight loss specifically, but also about changing, being happy, achieving, communicating and more. They're all part of the same advice really because until you understand more fully why you do what you do, how can you permanently adopt new behaviours? Information won't change your life. It can help you in understanding yourself and how then to take action in order to make the difference ... this time ... permanently, for ever, and for always.

But I'll tell you something, it is possible. Get the right combination of factors together and it's dynamite in your hands. You know you're the same as me, in many ways. Some may be more pronounced, others less marked. A variation on a theme. Or maybe a carbon copy of where I've come from and what I've been through, which is why I've just included so much of my story so you can see how similar you are to me. And therefore why you can trust me enough to give this system your all. So now I can be your soul mate. Join me here in a better frame of mind - with a greater understanding - having put the wheel in motion to help things change for the better - permanently. We just have to do it!

Chapter Twelve - This Whole Identity Thing

Powerful visualisations - reclaim your natural birthright to be slim!

What makes a woman accept being fat as a part of life? Is it because of the way she's treated? Is it because of what she's told by those around her? Is it because she's basically given up, that she has such a lack of self-worth that she puts up with being less than she deserves to be? Or just that she's kidding herself. How many times do we hear from people who've said that the final straw was "that photo at the barbecue, with butter running down my chin." Or "at the wedding where you couldn't see the bride because as maid of honour I blocked the aisle", or was it someone's comments? Those people who've become slim who still act like they're fat. The way they walk, dress, speak, or their confidence, their beliefs about food. They still comment on everyone else's eating habits, and obviously still have a huge hang-up about the whole food thing. They're in food prison, and unless they constantly exercise extreme self-deprivation and control, you just know that one day they're destined to be fat again - to once more grow into the body that fits the image they never grew out of in their mind.

There are also a few fat people who have so much confidence and who are not in food prison, and who grew up with a whole different set of rules surrounding food. Sure, they may like to be slimmer if they could tick a box, but quite frankly they feel ok as they are. Just go to the United States and your average slightly tubby person will feel positively slim comparatively speaking. There are just so many more much larger people there, unless you're in some parts of California, that even fourteen pounds or so overweight isn't considered unusual. Not that that helps the ones in food prison, nor does it help the likes of you and me when all we've got as a comparison is our own self-image - this year's model, last year's, the year before, but it's food for thought.

Visualisations

I'm going to take you on a journey into your mind. It's not hypnotism, or anything weird. It's just a basic way of installing a set of images which will help your mind get used to the idea that you can be slim. You can change. One of the biggest driving forces in a human being is the need to be consistent to your own identity, what you believe about who you really are. The dialogue you have about yourself. The words you use, the questions you ask yourself. These visualisation techniques can open up a new realm inside your mind, one where the slim you lays in hiding. Kept there by the resistance to change. It's not just a new wardrobe we're talking about here, it's having to give up all those excuses about your life. Like the woman who, every time she gets close to having to get on with her own life, or face up to sorting out a marriage gone wrong, hides behind having yet another baby. She doesn't really want another baby, in truth she just doesn't want to have to go back to being just herself again. So it is with the permanently fat person. Here's some food for thought. Think of how overweight you are. Are you usually the same number of pounds overweight? If you manage to keep yourself overweight by a few pounds, it's for a reason.

If you're always overspending the same proportion, no matter what your salary, if you're always late by the same amount of minutes each time, if your house / flat / room is always about the same degree of 'messy', then you're perpetuating certain beliefs about yourself which keep you at that level. Otherwise you'd go far higher wouldn't you? Chances are, most of the time, you'll be overweight by roughly the same amount. When you're not dieting, and you are 'too fat' by about twenty pounds all the time, it implies that you are capable of maintaining your weight at the same level, you just haven't worked out how to do it at the level you prefer, slightly lower on the scales. If someone isn't yet ready for the change to a slimmer image, nothing will help them. If you stay adamant that "it won't work for me," then guess what, it won't.

I'll keep saying it, one of the biggest driving forces in mankind is to stay consistent with your own identity. Studies which have been done on this subject show that in general, a person will fight harder not to change than to make change happen. We find it almost impossible to shake our old identity free. We want consistency and certainty. We've been down the route of being fat before and we're used to it. We've got all our fat clothes, our fat lifestyles, our excuses for not walking too far, or for not having a man. We know our fat image like a comfort blanket and we're sticking to it. We like our comfort zones. We prefer the status quo.(10)

Making things different is hard to cope with, which is why forming new habits is so much harder than breaking old ones. The first four weeks of the new fitness routine, or giving up smoking, or getting those essays done on time and so much more. They're all much harder than the twenty fourth week, or the eleventh month, or the sixtieth year. So what can we do to help ourselves accept a new identity and act accordingly? Lots of things and visualisations especially, can help enormously, as a part of the overall transformation.

Imagine yourself in twenty years' time. What if you've never changed those habits? What if you've stayed in food prison? What if all your photos, and video tapes from all those holidays in all those years had you looking the way you don't want to look fat (according to you at least)? I'll say 'fat' because there will be some of you who make everyone sick because you look great but just think you're fat. Others would die to look just like you, but nevertheless, you perceive yourselves to have a food problem, to not be able to eat normally. Perhaps the only reason you are decent looking to other people is because you've taken up permanent residence in food prison and refuse to come out. You've thrown away the key. But little do you realise that you could still keep your shape, even lose a little more maybe, if you gave up this addictive identity - this habit - and put something else in its place. If you formed new associations. New associations with your shape. A few pounds or a little roll around your middle is not "I'm fat". If you formed new associations with your eating habits and with other people's eating habits and with food in general, you would be given the key to a much happier life. And as for the rest of you who probably, or definitely, are fat, well imagine this, let your mind really run riot with this one for at least five minutes and get your feelings down on paper if you can.

Imagine if you had the key out of this food prison now; this year or even this month. Someone somewhere is going to come and teach you how to be a slim person and how to eat like one, think like one and act like one. Release yourself and those around you from all the hangups that food prisoners base their lives around. Would you pay big bucks for it? You bet you would! It would be on the bestseller list immediately.

Isn't that why so many so-called wonder cures, miracle-diets, latest food fads, diet trends, pills, potions, lotions, machines, operations, books, clubs, courses and diet foods are always so popular. But they never work permanently. What kind of industry is this that deals solely with the symptoms of a problem, and never truly get to grips with what's stopping it from providing a permanent solution? How many new diet books were released and sold last year, the year before and the decade before that? If you kept taking your car to a garage for the same repair over and over again in the course of your life, and every time you questioned what they were doing they blamed your driving, you'd begin to wonder if the garage really knew what it was doing, wouldn't you? You bet you would. Well it's the same with the diet industry. So you need never blame yourself again - ever - for not sticking to that rigid diet you swore blind was going to be the last ever one, because they don't work permanently. Think, dieting is now believed to actually lower your metabolic rate so much that your body then needs even fewer calories than it did before in order to reach the point at which it starts storing them up as fat. **So dieting can actually make you fatter**. Your body was born with a genetically predetermined bone structure, ideal weight and height distribution. Your predetermined weight is called your *set point*. Your body goes to great lengths to defend this designed weight, which is your *ideal body weight* - not your ideal, but your body's, whether you like it or not. Your body makes it very difficult to lose below this weight and very difficult to gain above this weight. It does this by raising or lowering your basal metabolism, which is the rate your body burns calories while at rest.(11) Dieting can reduce the metabolic rate by 15% - 40%, whereas forced feeding can increase the rate in some people as much as 75%. In one study, volunteers were fed double their usual intake over a six-month period, with the goal of increasing their weight by 20% - 25%. Although the first few pounds were gained easily, the total weight gained was 75% less than expected, based on intake, due to the fact that their metabolic rate increased. (11)

We all know what to do. We just don't do what we know. It's the 'why' that this is all about. So how can the visualisation help? Why don't you start with some me-time. I want you to find some soft music - background music, not strong melodies - and give yourself five minutes of 'me-time'. Get a pen and notebook, a journal style one if possible, in order to keep all your thoughts together. As Anthony Robbins says, "If your life's worth living, it's worth recording." (12) I agree, just don't get all anal about it. There's nothing worse than the feeling that you 'have to' do something. If you don't want to, don't do it! On the other hand, if you find you want to write for four hours and fill it front to back, then feel free to do that too: Freedom Living, remember? The great thing is, this bit is just for you. No one else will need to see it or read it unless you want them to. You may want to show someone special in order to help you make it more real - it's your call.

Now with the music playing, just write. Don't think about it too much, or stop, or think what you should be writing, just write, and get to the bottom of what it's really like to be fat. Your life, now. How does being fat hold you back, embarrass you, stop you from fulfilling your potential? Feel it, live it, write it. Visualise and record all this then you can *change it*. Write as much as you feel is inside you. Have some tissues ready just in case it all gets a bit emotional. For some people it will, for some it won't, there's no right or wrong, ok?

Ok, when you've done that, for now, think yourself forward whilst you're in this mode. What's life going to be like in five years' time if you don't make the changes? How will it affect your life, and the people around you? What will you miss out on? Now it gets even more intense. Think yourself forward ten years to what your life will be like if you haven't made the changes. Keep the music going, the same music for all of this thinking forward bit. You'll need a different more uplifting bit in a minute. I think you can guess what's coming. When you're right in the middle of visualising you in twenty years' time - the worst of it, if you never made the changes, I want you to make the first change and as soon as you're finished and ready for the next stage, change the music over.

Now remember, everything can be different, it's not too late. It's just like someone's given you another chance at the next twenty years. None of what you described has happened yet. You've got the opportunity to make a difference, if it starts right now. So now describe what you would be like - in the present initially, if you did start to make the changes you know are needed. Don't leave out any details. What would you feel like, how would people react differently to you. How confident would you be? Put it all down.

Now do the same again - for five and then ten years' time and think - how different would your life be? Fill yourself with that joyous feeling that you'd get if you knew it was all going to happen, and now do one last thing. Notice all the conditionals in what you've just written - should, would, could, if. Now I want you to re-write it as if it was true right now. As if your fairy godmother had wafted in with her wand and her hobnail boots and instantly given you your desires. "I am slim and beautiful. I am fit and active. I use the stairs instead of the lift. I walk the dog every morning before work. I never overeat. I always listen to my body. I am a size twelve skirt." If you want, these can be affirmations, or incantations, or your own code of conduct, whatever you want to call it. There are many different perceptions of this process. Louise Hay and Bernie Siegel talk about affirmations in their work.(13) Good old Tony Robbins calls the future you technique, The Dickens Process (ghosts of xmas future, present and past), and goes into this method more fully at his excellent *Unleash the Power Within /Life Revolution* weekends around the world, including at Wembley in London, Frankfurt in Germany and in the US, where you also get the chance to do a firewalk - I've done two now and they are wonderful metaphors for overcoming the barriers in your beliefs. Otherwise his books and tapes give lots more detail as to how these and other techniques can help you in your transformation.[(14)] Use it if it works for you too.

And if you're a real old-school sceptic, a cynic of the first degree, then do whatever part of this feels comfortable to you. Opening up your mind to some of the latest psychology can in itself be a giant leap and not one you can make readily or instantly, so again, don't worry about it. I only ask you to test the theory not necessarily to instantly believe. And if you can change the way you feel about your image, your identity, your self-belief and references, then you may have to think about who you are and what you stand for. Even if it's only a tiny change you make every time you sit down to think about it, then all those little changes will soon add up to be a big change, and you'll definitely be taking yourself onto a different path.

Do you know the best thing about Food Freedom? It's just this - it's allowing you to **reclaim your natural birthright to be slim**. Now go back into your past. If you can remember a time when you had no thought of food and were a normal weight, and you didn't worry about food the whole time, even if you occasionally considered cutting down a bit, or were conscious that you shouldn't eat too much chocolate in one go, then you are one of the lucky ones. Anyone can go back to the state you were born in, being able to naturally control what food your body needed to eat. You just have to do one thing. One thing. It's a big one.

Trust your body.

It doesn't come naturally, but it's something, which once you've started doing, will be as easy as breathing. Because it makes sense. Because it's not contrived. Because it's not depriving yourself. Because it's not going to make you get bored with it. Because it's not hard. Because it makes food even more enjoyable than it ever was before in your life. Because you see results. Because it's liberating. Because let's face it, it's easy. Babies can do it and toddlers can do it, if they haven't already been indoctrinated by contrived socialisation. Deprivation and control can kick in from a very early age, just look at some of the obese pre-school kids.

It's all gone wrong mainly in the last few hundred years, but more particularly, to be affecting those of us alive now, since the second world war. Rationing mentality has never really gone away. No wonder, if it's an intrinsic and powerful part of our child-rearing and has therefore become part of everyday life for us. And if it's good enough for us, it's got to be good enough for our children. Why does it perpetuate itself so much? Because we don't learn how to be parents from anyone else but those who bring us up. So what they do, by and large, we do. Oh sure, the brand of nappy, and the toys and pastimes may evolve, but why would it ever occur to you to change the habits we teach regarding food and mealtimes, when we don't even realise they're wrong? For decades now, we've been propounding the same myths to do with food and eating. Telling ourselves, and our children, the same stories. Even now, as I sit here in a hotel in Spain with my laptop, writing this chapter, the words I heard at lunchtime are resounding in my ears. My son left two potato croquettes on his plate. He'd finished. For me, that's a reason to rejoice! My mum's partner Tom, however, hasn't got it yet.

- *"Why don't you eat those other two, Brad? No point leaving them."*

- *"I've finished,' says Brad."*

- *"But there's only two, they're only small, eat them, they're lovely."*

- *"No."*

End of conversation. Thank goodness. My son is now in the world of the slim people. And though he may at times stuff himself with Maltesers and eat four packets of crisps, he is in touch with his body as much as the next slim person.

My daughter's just told me, since we're having this conversation, that daddy still asks her to finish what's on her plate! When they were out having a meal the other day, she told him, "I don't feel like it," and he replied, "Oh rubbish!" Ever heard that one before? Ever done that one before? How on earth anyone can second guess what another person feels is beyond me! He should definitely know better by now. But he'll get used to it. As Wayne Dyer says to the people who try to insist he acts as they want him to act. “You want me to do it your way? You think I'm wrong? You'll get over it.”[(11)]

The best thing we can do for our children is never comment on body shapes or criticise their eating in relation to a part of their anatomy. The days of, "What are you eating that for, you'll get fat as an old pig," have long ceased to be a problem for me. It still amuses me somewhat that my mother will still say, "What are you eating now?" But if I just remind myself that it usually happens when she's back at slimming club and is feeling the deprivation and control more markedly than usual, it helps me recognise the place she's in, and just let it go. The need for retribution is useless in the quest to understand your own body and its foibles, and smiling sweetly and just acknowledging the critic's comments can often get the message across more effectively than ever trying to waste time explaining it all, or worse - arguing. Vikki told me at the start of all this that other people will learn when they are ready, and there's no point trying to get them into the Freedom Eating ethic until they want to know. Never a truer word. I have had great success with my sister, who now seems to understand the principles behind it a little more, but is presently some way off from true Food Freedom.

But she'll get there - when she's ready and she will join the thousands around the world finally breaking free from food prison into a brave new world. Ironically, the same world we would have lived in our entire lives, had social conditioning and learned behaviour, habits and deprivation and control not interfered.

So once you've mastered the art of changing your own image of yourself and not living up to the expectations of those around you who may put you off, you will be ready to help those people when they see the change in you and want some of it for themselves. They'll be ready for Food Freedom.

Chapter Thirteen - Food Freedom in a Nutshell

How you can finally get out of food prison - just do it!

The first thing you have to do is to let go. Let go of all the rules you've ever learned surrounding food. You know the ones: I mustn't eat now, I must eat this before that, and not too much of that. I can fill up on vegetables, however tasteless and stress making they may be. I can't have 'bad' foods, or I'm being bad. I must be 'good' and comment on everyone else's eating habits too, to help me deal with my own inability to feed my body just what it needs, in the right quantity, at the right time.

The first thing I want you to do on this programme is sit and write a little list of what you would be like if you stopped being controlled by food, or overeating a little but too often. It's genie of the lamp time - three wishes can be yours - the body and life you desire. Right now. Let your imagination run riot. What would you look like? How would you feel? What would you wear? How would others react to you? In which situations?

Writing all this down, and in fact, keeping a little bit of a journal about your transformation will really help you remember how far you've come. Pretty soon, it will become so natural for you to eat normally, you'll forget ever being any different. So do give yourself some me-time and write. Keep it safe. You'll need it later.

Now get out those photos. The ones you hoped would never see the light of day. The ones where some horrid fatty has taken you over, and possessed your body. You were going along quite happily, doing the same thing for years and years, and then all of a sudden there in the minor was this plump person, and you didn't like what you saw. You're not one of the tiny minority of perfectly happy fat people who don't mind being that size, and that's fine for them, but not for you. So get out those photos, and make a little album if you want. Or if it's all been too much for you in recent times, and you haven't even allowed any pics to be taken of you, get cracking straight away. Take some from the most unflattering angles, wearing the most unflattering clothes. Just imagine being able to take a photo of this fat person in the lens, and know that they are on their way out - their control over you and your appearance, and your inability to get into that little black number from a couple of

Christmases ago, is all about to go for good. *It's about to end. Your journey is about to begin.*

1- Only eat when you're physically hungry.

This is not as easy to do, or as obvious as you may think. Many of us will eat because we think we're hungry, but actually, we're really thirsty. Or we're hungry for something else other than food, like company or a hug or some physical activity. So how do you know? When you're really hungry, there is no doubt about what you want. I want you to get to the stage where you absolutely know every time, without a shadow of doubt, that you are physically hungry. What are the signs your body gives you to say it's time to eat? And it doesn't have to just be hunger pangs in your stomach. The signs it's time to eat are:

-People will get a little bit ratty.

-Some a little bit faint.

-Some will get the beginnings of a headache.

-Some a little bit irrational, with a slight feeling of panic.

-Often you will just be thirsty, so have a glass of water and then if you still have the feeling fifteen minutes later, you are definitely hungry.

-On a scale of one to ten, you're definitely at six or above.

Sometimes you will wander around the kitchen not able to make up your mind what it is you want to eat. That means you're almost definitely not hungry. Have some water instead - seriously, it can be as simple as that. You'll get to know after a while if it is. After fifteen minutes, if the feeling's still there, then work out what that feeling actually means. It could be any number of body hungers just crying out to be satisfied; from loneliness to boredom, frustration to anger, we feed each of them with food.

This is what we call comfort eating. And we don't need to do it. It's ok to stand firm and refuse to give in. We cannot go to the kitchen and distract ourselves with food. We can leave it. But you must turn your attention to whatever else is it that your body is hungry for. What's it telling you? Start getting in tune with the messages - fundamentally, they may feel like a call for food, but you think that out of habit. They are really subtly different calls for different needs. A hug may be all you need to satiate that hunger signal your body is sending out. It'll be misty at first, but with practice, the signals become clear, and believe me, getting this one right will be a major step towards a happier you.

Don't wait Too Long.

But equally, don't wait too long. If hungry is good, then starving is not better. If you leave it too long, say, till you're on a ten on the hunger scale, then you'll be too ravenous to notice the subtle changes that imply it's time to stop now, and as you *inhale* your food, you go way past the point of being satisfied, you're almost certain to overeat. That's still ok, and don't beat yourself up but you'll know next time not to leave it so long before listening to what your body's trying to tell you.

Particularly when you get into Food Freedom proper, you will almost certainly find you're eating little and often. This is also being taught now as a way of increasing your metabolic rate. There's a lot of research around, backing up the nutritionists who are saying eat five or six smaller meals every day and that's intrinsically part of Food Freedom for many of us. Around a fistful of food every time is often all it takes to go from hunger to satisfaction, although this is not a rule. There are no rules, only guidelines, and if you wish to overeat and ignore the signals and the guidelines on certain occasions, then you have to know that that's also all right occasionally. As is learning to stop long before you used to. After years of indoctrination that we're supposed to clear our plates. It's so liberating to leave some. Try it, it's ok, you're allowed.

But then don't feel something's wrong if you find yourself needing to eat again only a short while later. It could be you're now hungry for exactly the same foods as you were earlier on, and there's nothing wrong in that either. So, if you'd kept some of the earlier meal, you could quite easily just finish off what you left at the last meal, and believe me, when you're hungry again later, the take away box with the rest of your restaurant meal will be just as exquisite as it was the first time.

2- Only eat till you're satisfied, not till you're full.

This is probably the biggest error we all make in our progress towards obesity. We've been taught to override our bodies' signals all our lives, so no wonder it starts to go wrong on us, and creates the never ending spiral towards a bigger body with each new diet, fad or temporary regime, however permanent we tell ourselves we meant it to be this time.

To be satisfied, you

-Should not be able to feel the food in your stomach.

-Should aim to consume around a fistful in size every sitting.

-May get a sudden deep breath (this is my biggest sign nearly every time), as if your body's saying, "ahhh, that's better, thank you."

-Will almost certainly notice the food change in degree of tastiness. It stops having the 'oh wow' factor. It will still taste good, but not fantastic. You can stop now - try a few times. If you're a real food lover, this technique is brilliant, it means you're only ever eating when the food tastes unbelievably fantastic, because you stop when that taste explosion ends. When the food changes flavour from being outstanding to just good, or even just ok, that's when your body's had enough of that flavour. Try something else, and if it all begins to taste like cardboard, your body is no longer in need of that food anymore. It's satisfied. If in any doubt, leave it fifteen minutes and try again, try the thing you like the look of on the plate most.

3- Give the food your full attention.

Literally do nothing else at the same time as eating. Don't read, don't drive, don't watch TV. Heck, in the first few weeks, don't even have a conversation with anyone, and always sit down. If you must be a fridge picker, at least pull up a chair and do it. This is without a doubt one of the most important guidelines in order to listen to your body and its subtle signals. Remember, hunger shouts but satisfaction whispers. If you're distracted by something and not paying full attention, you will miss out on the full enjoyment of that food and as a result, feel a little deprived. You might possibly miss those subtle signals that your body's had enough and it's time to stop.

4- Think about what your body really needs, not what your brain really wants..

Eat what your body wants the most. This is one of the most important guidelines too, and they're all just guidelines, not rules. If your body is giving you a message, it's for a reason. So if a basic omelette cries out to you from the menu at the classy restaurant, but you'd usually choose steak to make it 'worthwhile being there', go with the body's needs and choose the omelette. Chances are your body will enjoy it so much more, the taste explosion will be reward in itself, as your taste buds for some reason respond much more intensely to the flavours your body really really needs, be it smoked salmon and scrambled egg, or Caesar salad - without the chicken even though you're not usually vegetarian. Just trust in your body and go with the flow.

5- You can do this even if you're on a diet.

If you're on a diet at this stage, just choose accordingly from the *allowed* menu. If you desperately can't get rid of your need for rules and a structured format, if you've spent too many years mistrusting your own body so that you daren't put it back in charge straight away, don't worry. The whole point of Food Freedom is that you should feel free to do what feels right, and if part of that for you right now is to follow a diet plan, just use the guidelines above within your framework of counting things. The idea is that you'll be giving your body the chance to eat more the way nature intended without the artificial habits we've accumulated over the years from our peers and from so-called experts. For instance, "fill up on vegetables." Why? Stop when your body feels comfortable, no matter what's left on the plate. No matter how many calories or points you've got left to use up that day. No matter if the diet says it's a free food. Why stuff it down your throat if your mouth tells you it's tasteless and therefore it's had enough of it? The subtle nuances of taste are one of the most enjoyable clues to successful Food Freedom. Plus wait till you're body hungry, always remember that.

And when you begin to like this new feeling of your body responding to its messages, when you finally feel you can learn to trust it again, that's when you can truly start choosing whatever the hell you want to eat, even if it's the most fattening clotted cream and Devon scone imaginable because you'll probably only eat some of it anyway. With practice, this system just starts to make so much sense. Eventually you may be able to progress on to full freedom, which is:

6- If you want something 'bad', go ahead and eat it. Or maybe if during one meal, you end up overeating slightly, just don't beat yourself up about it afterwards.

Now remember, we're only eating between hunger and satisfaction, so our body will be able to tell us to stop whenever it's had enough. And we're giving it our full attention, so we remember every single morsel, none has been devoured by the 'cookie monster', the one that takes all your cookies when you're too busy watching the film to notice you've actually eaten them all yourself. We've all done that one. Even the smallest portion, one or two chips, one square of chocolate, one glass of wine - have been your downfall in the past. You've broken the diet, and since you're in food prison, then you binge as a result. The Last Supper syndrome can only slip in when you hand yourself over to it. So if you stop feeling bad after doing it, you're less likely to take it to the point of no return. Never punish yourself again. This psychological distinction is so powerful. For those of us who want something much more whenever we know we can't have it, this may be the turning point in your escape from food prison. No food is outlawed and no food is a trigger for beating yourself up. We all know we eat these foods from time to time anyway, we just call it being 'bad', so why not take away the mystique and desirability by saying it's no longer out of bounds? Give them equal value with other food, and that means you can have anything you like. If :

- *You're genuinely hungry.*

- *Your body really wants it.*

- *You can give it your full attention.*

- *You listen to your body and stop when you're satisfied and that means stopping before you can feel the food in your stomach.*

Give yourself permission. Making these foods allowed removes the chance of triggering off a binge or a Last Supper. And if you do occasionally go past satisfaction, learn from it, let it go, move on, and adjust next time. After all, the answer to over eating is just wait till you're hungry before eating again.

Slim people may have a milkshake too much at one mealtime, then eat less for the rest of the day. Serial dieters will have the milkshake then eat more for the rest of the day. It's all a matter of trust, because it's all in the mind and here's where you must start trusting your body. It's all a matter of trust. You're not going to change overnight, but each time and every time you try it, you get nearer to doing it permanently and naturally. In the end, you'll find over eating becomes alien to your body.

7 - Be an observer, not a judge.

The observer says "I just had a little too much mashed potato, and now I feel a little too full. Hmm, that's interesting, I wonder why I did that?" The observer may even come up with a few suggestions as to why you did it, which will help you for next time. The judge in you, on the other hand, will shoot you down in flames, remind you of the last twenty or thirty times you did exactly the same thing, and call you the pits of the earth for letting yourself down - again! Just let go of the whole food prison thing, which includes discussing the rights and wrongs, the goods and the bads and playing the guilt game.

One of the most liberating parts of Food Freedom is letting go of the need to comment, to criticise those around you and their eating habits, as well as your own. How wonderful not to have to play the role of food monitor ever again, and start losing weight at the same time? The loss will not be instant, even though some people, who have obviously completely screwed up their eating patterns over the years, do report substantial losses in the early weeks, once they get back to a more natural way of feeding their bodies just the fuel they need to live.

A tiny difference every day will lead you to your destination in the end.

You make a tiny difference every day to your habits of a lifetime and all the little differences will gradually add up. A golfer correcting a golf swing or a helicopter pilot using the ultra sensitive joystick controls will make the tiniest adjustment this end, to see a big impact on the outcome. The golf ball sent a fraction of a degree more to the left at the tee will end up much further over to the left two hundred yards down the line. And that's where I want you to end up. Seeing a big difference in months to come, as a result of little changes now. Start gently, and keep re-reading this book till it all sinks in. This is not a quick fix.

You continue your search for an instant answer, a drastic solution, and you'll never earn your 'get out of jail free' card. But just start using parts of this method - the ones that make the most sense to you right now, even if you can't do it all straight away. Sometimes it takes a long time to give up the habits of a lifetime, and that's understandable. Whatever you choose to do will be right for you right now. What I'm not going to do is get all heavy on you and demand you follow rules. I want this book to be your little helper, your little inspiration. Keep referring back to it, even when you don't feel you're doing it right, and eventually you'll feel ready to persevere, when the time is right for you. Then the little differences you're making now will make permanent changes down the line.

If you're a person perpetually watching your weight, suddenly converting to absolutely no calorie counting or points watching is a terrifying prospect. So don't worry about it. Do what feels good to you now, and let this book be a little haven of hope in the sea of diet plans you've sailed in for so long, and whenever the crossing gets a little bit too stormy for you, then re-read this book, or the parts you really like, the ones that touch a nerve or hit home, and try again. Never say Food Freedom didn't work for you. If it doesn't work, you're just not ready to give up deprivation and control, and to start trusting your body. Not just yet anyway. You will be ready to do it wholeheartedly one day. Until then, do what you can, and that will be enough - for now. (*2014 note – or do The 'When' Diet element alongside other traditional methods.)*

The same goes for exercise. Now there are people who swear by exercise to get results for their body, and others who can't stand it. All I'm going to say is if it feels good, you'll do it. Exercise is vital for all of us to live longer, healthier lives. We all know it. It's just getting ourselves to do it that's the problem. *Deja vu?* Well yes, the similarities between making ourselves eat more normally and making ourselves do exercise are endless, and you can add to the list, making ourselves stop smoking, stop drinking, stop taking drugs, stop being argumentative and much more. We know what we should be doing, it's just making ourselves do it.

It's all a state of mind.

If you can find a way of making it enjoyable, of making it the natural choice, of making it your best friend, that's when you'll do it on a regular basis. With exercise in particular, I'd urge you to find something you can do easily that gives you pleasure. It could be buying a dog and walking it every day. It could be playing badminton with a friend. It could be sex. Whatever works for you. That's always the key - whatever works for you. Experts like Ayurvedic metaphysics lecturer, Deepak Chopra's views on enough exercise are well worth finding out about. For example in Magical Body, Magical Mind, he says a bit of yoga, a bit of brisk walking, regularly, or the like, are much more likely to help you get it into your lifestyle on a regular basis than forcing yourself to commit to a tough gym regime, or extreme workout, which you do for a while then stop, and go back to doing nothing.[16] Honestly, check it out, it's great reading, or listening if you get the audio version. But basically, walking the dog is a great way of just getting started. Or set yourself a trip to walk each day, down to get the paper instead of having it delivered, a more distant sandwich shop at lunchtime, round to see a friend using the pram instead of the car to take the baby out. However, you need to check with you GP before starting any new exercise regime.

And stretching every day is one of the very best ways of just feeling better long term. Too many headaches or shoulder pains could be avoided or helped if you only did something different with your muscles every day instead of the same old sitting, standing, sleeping routine. Our bodies were made to move. Only in recent centuries have our lives become more inactive. Even our lymphatic system in our body doesn't have a pump to make it circulate because we were evolved to get it moving by exercising. So move we should, if we can, as long as it works for us and not if it doesn't, and there are all sorts of programmes and systems to follow if you want to get more fun into it, or if you want to get specialised too.

THE EGOSCUE METHOD - for postural training. This is an amazing system I've been using myself to help correct problems with my alignment. A bit like Callanetics crossed with Pilates, but with very precise motions and it is superb for toning and it really works.

DANCE VIDEOS - I know it might sound silly, but use all the usual dance and aerobic videos, as these are fun. Just jig around in your lounge, learning some of the routines to some of the latest pop songs. Great!

A YOGA VIDEO - that's varied enough not to be boring, but rigorous enough to work includes relaxation, detox and deep breathing.

FACIAL EXERCISES - with Eva Fraser, a lovely lady. I did a few hours with her on QVC and have done a few of her exercises most days ever since. She's over seventy but looks in her fifties, and it's genuine. It doesn't take long, and makes a great gift for someone if you need an excuse for sampling it first.

FARADIC EXERCISES - all have their place in toning and motivating you, with limited applications, but you do see results if you use them right. The lovely Anita Harris can vouch for their efficacy.

EXERCISE MACHINES - if you really want a recommendation, then I'd say go for an elliptical cross trainer. It's like being on a bike but you're standing and most use upper body as well. This is just my preference, other people may prefer different types. And I find ab-trainers are excellent for targeting the stomach muscles, and again, you don't need hours on them to see a bit of a result, particularly if you use them regularly - same old story, you see. Mustn't forget the Pilates Performer either. Many of these are available from shopping telly if you can't find them in the shops.

Basically, just see if you can do a bit of something every day. Because remember the increments rule, if you make a one per cent difference every day, then you've made a thirty per cent difference by the end of just one month.

8- Don't set yourself up to fail by having too many rules. Forget every rule surrounding food.

That's the fundamental key to food freedom. Freedom living is about going with the flow. By not setting yourself up for failure by making your targets too high. Why should a successful day consist of not having eaten any fat, run five miles, sorted the kids out, done a bit of housework, paid a few bills, rung your mum, and had a fruitful day at work? Add to that little concoction, making mad passionate love and remembering to exfoliate and you really are on a hiding to nothing.

The food rules are the bars of our prison. They are the veil through which we view the world. We've imprisoned ourselves with foodie rules since the time of rationing.

9- Listen to how your body responds to the food in your stomach and learn how to make a good match. Learn to trust your body.

This is probably the most important guideline to true freedom. Don't underestimate it! If you can possibly start off by doing a little food/mood diary at the beginning of your quest to Food Freedom, it will help give you a better understanding of what works for your body and what doesn't.

There's a lot to be said for food combining. But read a book like *The Diet Cure* by Julia Ross, and you may find other combinations apart from the Hay ones that work best for your body. Then follow Living Health by Anthony Robbins [11.] We all know about the trend for food and diet fads, and what's fashionable and a must now, may change in a few years, so why was it right in the first place? Well you can end all that, by just listening to your body. Of course, this is not medical advice, still check with your relevant expert for any serious concerns, but the basics should hold up for most people. Once you've eaten that meal, be a scientist experimenting on your own body, and record or note the effects afterwards. Then make the appropriate changes and try it again, and keep trying till you get a winning combination, and the exciting thing? No experiment was wasted - you can't get it wrong- you're just ruling out one more type of food experience not to repeat in the same way in the future, or at least by choosing it you'll be well aware of what it will do to you!

Observing the results of each meal on your body is the ultimate key to freedom. Please do it! No freedom eater is ever truly happy and free unless they listen to their body afterwards. As Vikki says, "We may not know exactly why it works, but it works." Maybe later you'll discover the science behind the result. Maybe you won't, but at least you'll be living in the world of the slim people and will have found something you can stick with at long last. So try it.

10- Don't forget the water thing.

This is a personal crusade of mine, and one I've added to the Food Freedom basics, after my studies on water and its effect on the body. In particular new types of water now available.[18] Too many of us are dehydrated, we need to give our bodies the means to carry out all those electrical functions going on inside our organs, in our minds, in our lungs. Most of the activity inside us is the result of little neuro peptides connecting with other cells across a gap containing fluids. If there's not enough fluid around these cells, then they're not going to perform as efficiently. You're not going to concentrate as well, and if you're up working late, needing to think straight and you're drinking too much tea or coffee, not only are you flooding your body with caffeine, which is a drug, but you're also extracting fluids out of your cells, because these drinks are diuretics. So drink more water, throughout the day. Don't forget the guidelines: drink, in ounces, half what your body weighs in pounds (14lb to a stone, 16 fl oz to 500ml). So for example, a 140 lb woman may need 70 oz of water a day, that is approximately four and a half pints or two and a half litres. Roughly three litres a day for most people. So maybe you'll be ok to drink the coffee after dinner, but not on an empty stomach unless you have a full glass of water first, or after, or both. Get to listen to your body and trust it.

If you've gone on a diet where you can have unlimited fizzy drinks and caffeine (black tea or coffee), or even unlimited salads or veg, and you've used them to excess, no wonder you've felt bad. Now according to the diet, that's ok, but your body's sending you warning signals that it's not happy - a headache, feeling dizzy or hyper, queasiness maybe. So if you've still got the diet mentality, don't be a sheep and inflict someone else's rules on your body.

Find out what worked for you and write your own guidebook. You're unique, and your body could be unique too.

11- Keep listening.

Vikki knows she can eat some sweets and puddings as long as she has a bit of protein as well. When I read *The Diet Cure*, by Julia Ross, it seems there's a precise reason why this makes sense, to do with insulin, glycogen and the pancreas. Now Vikki didn't know this, but her body did. This may work for you too, or it may not. We can never say the rules will be identical for all of us. We're all different blood types, and everyone has unique DNA, so why should our food requirements be uniform? Another reason why diet sheets with set menus don't work long-term. Talking of blood groups, maybe you'll have followed the 'Eat Right for your Type' guidelines or maybe you're fascinated with the ayurvedic beliefs regarding doshas.

We're all different body types, eg, Vata, Pitta or Kapha, and therefore have different requirements. Their advice has worked for you in the past, and it's all certainly very interesting, but just goes to underline the fundamental, crucial role of listening to your own body and finding out what's right for you. Nearly all these plans recommend drinking enough water. We have evolved, after all to drink plain water, for the vast majority of the hundreds and thousands of years which have taken us to where we are now on the evolutionary scale. Stone age man didn't have Starbucks or a drinks vending machine on every corner.

It's a learning procedure, and you're not usually going to do it perfectly the first few times you do it. It's like anything - the more you do it, the better you'll do it, the more natural it'll feel. Be patient. This is not a means to and end, this is an end in itself. If you're listening, then you're doing it right. Even if what you hear is that the last meal you ate was a mistake, you listened, and that's what counts - learn, and move on. Food Freedom leads to a slimmer body and a less angst-ridden lifestyle, they are the outcomes. It's not a quick fix, it's a farewell to all those years of misery and a final goodbye to thinking that you can starve yourself to achieve a permanent shape change. In the process, you may get much slimmer. That's a frequent result for users of this system over the last fourteen years or so, but the purpose of doing it is not to lose a stone, it's merely the 'doing it' itself. To finally break free from food prison, and to live in the world of the slim people. To consider yourself normal around food. Now that's the true freedom, and listening to your body will take you there.

12- Accept whatever shape and weight your body wants to be.

In the era of Twiggy, and more recently the supermodel waif look, even the most curvy women wanted to be straight up and down with no sign of flab anywhere. In the Renaissance period it was fashionable to be plump. Some of the figures in those paintings had rolls you could store your sandwiches in. But irrespective of fashion, if your body wants to be what you regard as half a stone overweight, then so be it. Or if your breasts finally surrender to gravity and do their best impression of floppy dogs ears, there's not a lot, bar surgery, you can do about it. But wouldn't you rather be a happier more content version of you than the one that's been driving you bonkers for the last God knows how many years, being miserable and thinking about food endlessly. Not much of a trade off, huh? Just adjust your expectations accordingly, a small price to pay for escaping food prison. Once you're a true Freedom Eater, you'll have a permanent passport into the land of the slim, being comfortable with who you are, not feeling the need to judge other people's choices of meal or comment on the drink they choose at the bar. After all, they didn't have you and your rules in mind when they chose it. End of story.

13- Don't let others, or your own thoughts, get you down.

Once you release yourself from the need to seek the approval of others, the world becomes a better place. To be independent of the good opinion of others doesn't mean go all out to be nasty or awkward and not care what they think.[19] Rather it frees you up to listen to you and work out what's the right thing for you. You know you better than anyone else, after all. Get to know you. Spend some time in your own company. Get to know your own mind. This might not work for everybody, but it does for me: meditate if you can - it's just a lovely way of doing a bit of daily relaxation. I love doing Transcendental Meditation, it's helped me deal with my tendency towards asthma over the years too, and although the sceptics may sniff, unless you look into it and actually find out more or maybe try it, you never know how something new may benefit you.

And if it's a mind thing - stress, worry, past experiences you keep reliving - listen, there are so many self-help, psychology and empowerment tapes and books out there, you can discover a whole new world if you just look into it. Check out more info on my website about books which help deal with various situations which can be the source of your comfort eating.

14-Stand guard at the door of your mind.

Most people operate from the same two fears:

1 - That they won't be loved.

2 - That they're not enough. They just don't measure up.

If either of those hits hard in your psyche, don't worry, you're not alone. And all I can say is listen to some of the best self-help tapes in order to take your mind and body to a new level of awareness. Go on a seminar. Do something new, with someone new. Take your brother out to lunch, or the friend you don't see and rarely speak to on the phone. Give yourself ammunition to fight back.

Your body will tend to try to stick to the old identity and remember that one of the strongest driving forces in the human personality is to be consistent with your existing identity, and if someone has decided they have a food problem, then a food problem they will have. They believe it, so it becomes, and stays, real for them. Morning noon and night. Every single day for the rest of their life. So why be like them? Make a stand for independence. Read new books, go new places, make new friends - ones who don't know the old you who talked about weight all the time. Or just start gradually changing. It can be an exciting challenge to yourself to deal with slowly introducing new changes in familiar situations. You decide to eat a cream cake in front of your mother, because you really really feel like one. Smile at her predictable reaction, but you don't need to rise to retaliation, because you're the one who's getting out of food prison, and she'll hopefully follow your example at a later date. But do it.

When you're out clothes shopping with your daughter, don't stand tutting at what's wrong with your body, start letting those feelings go. They don't have to be part of the new you, and maybe it won't be too late to help her avoid the pitfalls you've gone down your whole adult life as a result of re-enacting the sayings, phrases and beliefs your mum used to come out with in similar situations. And do you know? If you start that cream cake, and get criticised for it, when you then leave half of it because your body's had enough of it, and ask for a takeaway bag so you can enjoy the rest of it later, make a mental note of what your mum says then. A useful reply, (if you have to give one because explaining about Food Freedom isn't yet enough) is always Wayne Dyer's, "you'll get over it," accompanied by a big smile, of course. I do recommend his book and tape Pulling Your Own Strings.[(19)] It all helps. Anything to enhance the positive new identity you're building up for yourself the new you.

Talk to yourself every night about the new you. Or chant when you're jogging, or recite your new identity phrase in the car each morning after the school run. Do a bit of creative visualisation (eg in Shakti Gawain's book by the same name[(20)]) to imagine yourself in your new body. What a lovely feeling that will be to carry you through the day.

But don't hurry it, ok? Your body will do its stuff in its own time, and it may take longer if you've been messing around with it for so long. But it can take charge once more, and start giving out the signals again, and as long as you remain faithful and true to your trusty body, and listen, note and respond. It will come up trumps for you, eventually bringing you the shape you were meant to have. In the process you'll be achieving the behaviour you were meant to have around food. Permanently. Just give it time, and use your thought processes wisely in the meantime, not to beat yourself up, feel sorry for yourself or over-indulge in yet another Last Supper, but to find things to feel good about, and focus on. Whatever we focus on expands. Keep thinking you've got a weight problem and that's what will show up for you in your life, or start seeing yourself as being free of the old chains of food prison, and it'll happen all the faster for you. That's why these exercises and little challenges can really help you on your way.

Then when you hear that apparently we have about 60,000 thoughts every day and 95% of them are the same as yesterday, at least you'll know that by changing, expanding and growing, you're on the right path. Hang on in there because the journey can be a roller-coaster ride, but you'll love what's at the end of the line. Just keep at it. Whether you've reached the point of no return and have to do something about it now, or not. If you keep returning to diets, that's fine. Do what works for you, but I find you're only truly able to comprehend this amazing freedom - this transformation - if you do it all, wholeheartedly. It's your decision. You decide.

Chapter Fourteen - Binge Management

Breakthrough time! The system that recognises that we're human - this is your emergency routine!

If this is the first chapter you turn to, then you may be still in diet mode, you still have the diet mentality. Great, read on. This will be good. The next diet will be 'the one', won't it? Stick to it like glue will you? Lose all the weight? Keep it off permanently, right? Ok, fine. That's the place you're in right now and I know how it feels. I've been there too. Your next diet will work and you're not quite ready to let go of the habits of a lifetime and that's understandable. Whilst many can, some people can't. So keep this book as a standby. It's the 'break glass in emergencies only' handbook, ok? Tell you what, keep it just so you never have to use it. Like the 'fat day' outfit you keep in the back of the wardrobe 'just in case'.

Just in case you need it, here's your Food Freedom guide to binge management.

Of course you're not going to break this next diet - the one in the latest book - the one your best friend lost two stone on and kept it off, so far. But *just in case*, this is your Elastoplast to help cope with it. How about a method of having that chocolate / doughnut / fish and chips / pastry *without* needing to beat yourself up about it afterwards? For those 'you know you shouldn't' moments, when all else (reserve, willpower, logic, fat photos, tears, anger, torment, throwing up, tablets, disapproval, tut-tutting partner, minor), fails, use these guidelines to make sure you minimise the detour off the straight and narrow. **It is damage limitation and it works.**

It'll give you a sample of what Food Freedom is all about. During a binge, you've thrown away the diet rules anyway, so forget the diet rules and try this method. After all, you may like it so much, it becomes your new way of life instead of diet/ binge/ guilt/ binge/ diet - we know the routine. Read the whole book - if you want to for amusement only, or, for curiosity value. Or dip into it however you choose. Do whatever works best for you. Then pay particular attention to the detailed explanations for the sections mentioned in the advice I'm about to give you - there are more details on these topics throughout this book, but this is it in a nutshell for the serial browser - the one who has all the books under the sun and has 'done' each of them, but is still looking for the permanent solution. And if you never need it, this book can be a great present for someone else who does.

Binge Management - Damage Limitation

The Rules are driving you round the bend. You're at breaking point. Or you're just too down or emotional to diet today. Or you broke the diet and now you want to keep breaking it and eat the entire larder then start again tomorrow. STOP! Forget the usual pattern just this once - and do this instead, and for the first binge do all of this if you can. After that, just follow the main guidelines. There's also a lot more info on these topics in the rest of the book.

1. Take a breath and consider.

Pre-binge, just give yourself a second or two to consider what you're about to do. And I don't mean the usual berate yourself whilst still consuming the daily calorie requirement of a Canadian Lumberjack. I mean think about this place you're in. Give yourself a bit of 'me time'. Jot down a few sentences about how you got here - fast and furious - just get it all out on paper, whatever it is. Now take a breath. Literally - a deep breath. Several if possible. Stand up and stretch a bit - your neck, your back, your shoulders, more if possible. You're about to enjoy some wonderful flavours the decision's been made - so calm down, you don't have to panic. But you might need to move a little - your body's signals may be just giving you the sign for, "stretch me a bit please," and you're missing it amidst the imminent binge frenzy. It's me time, and you deserve it, so stretch out.

2. Now drink some water.

A big glassful if possible. If you're dehydrated you need it, if you're getting all anxious and hungry, chances are you may first and foremost be dehydrated. Dehydration is what commonly gives me the, "I gotta eat, I gotta eat" panic, but what it really means is, "water, for goodness sake!" You're going to eat something soon anyway, just give your body what it desperately needs first.

3. Now write down your binge list.

Write down in order, the binge foods you'd normally go for. What would you have right now, usually, and what effect would they have on your body? Abbreviate if necessary, but just think yourself through it for a second. Forget the diet, go from your past record do it from memory if you can. Perhaps the last binge was recent therefore easier to remember. One of mine might have looked something like the following, and i**f you still feel the overpowering urge to dive headlong into a binge, you just can't wait, go ahead, but try this technique next time.**

- Vanilla slice - fresh (sheer luxury - starving - tastes like heaven)

- Caramac bar - (childhood comfort connections).

- Low-fat crisps - (something savoury - not too high fat).

- Ryvita and low-fat cheese and cucumber, apple - (an attempt to balance it out).

- Milky Bar, the chunky kind - (tasted nice at first, then got less flavoursome very quickly indeed).

My stomach is starting to complain, I can feel the food in my stomach. The tastiness levels decline and I'm feeling guilty but not enough to stop. I'm starting to get to the 'vengeance' stage - taking revenge on myself for being so bad. I know I should stop right now and it won't be too bad. But my usual pattern is to now continue, partly in order to wreak revenge on my body for giving in and being weak, and anyway, I want more chocolate in my mouth.

- Twix - my favourite, usually. Although now I can't experience a chocolate 'high' as the hunger is all used up.

Taste buds pick up: "Yes, it's chocolate," rather than, "oh my God this is wonderful, how could I possibly live without this amazing taste in my mouth, I'm so enjoying this I wish I lived in a sweetshop."

Feeling fidgety. Still wanting to eat. Feeling appeased but not enough to stop. Torment, I know I should. But I don't want to. I've fed the feeling but it's still there. Maybe I should make it a big binge and go out and buy something else. Wait - haven't checked the freezer.

- Ice cream Snickers and it's hard work eating this one and by the end, I feel a sickly sweet feeling filling up my gullet.

I'm on a chocolate high. I feel a bit spaced out. I still feel fidgety. I try to concentrate on doing something else.

I resume previous activity but it doesn't last long, I head towards the biscuit tin.

- Bourbon biscuit, and I don't like Bourbons but they're the only thing in there. I eat half of one anyway. And I remember why I don't like them. I might have had too much chocolate. I will try something else to see if that does it, something nourishing maybe.

- Slimming chicken and rice meal for one. I hate to waste an expensive ready-made meal on a binge, but feel my body needs 'proper' food. Chicken rice, and a few vegetables - there, I have had vegetables. I can be virtuous. Everything tastes like cardboard. I leave a little and put it in the bin. Hah! I can control self and leave some food in the manner of a slim person instead of compulsively finishing the whole meal every time. I think it's over. I go back to activity. I definitely can't concentrate now as my stomach is distinctly uncomfortable, and in non-diet state. I sit feeling more and more angry with myself. I must really diet tomorrow. I will eat half my normal diet allowance to make up for today. I will be starving and the thought terrifies me, filled with dread at not getting food. Imminent famine and starvation and deprivation. PANIC!

- Other half of Bourbon

- Other bit of slimming meal for one from the bin! Shit! I am now truly disgusting. I have descended to the pits of the earth, along with other terrible people from history.

I have returned to the dreaded Willpower-Free Zone - it knows me only too well. It knows my weaknesses. It sends demons into my head enticing me with thoughts of even more sweet or high-calorie 'bad' food. I try no to succumb. I try diversionary tactics, whilst beating myself up continuously. I check my weight, just in case, on the off chance my metabolism has sped up mysteriously and eaten up all of the calories I've just consumed. I get on the scales. Aaahh! I have gone back up to what I was two weeks ago at the start of my diet. I get off, check the zero calibration and twiddle the knob. I try again. Aaahh! It's gone up another two pounds. I try the knob a few more times. The only acceptable result is when the starting position is minus five pounds. It must be my clothes so I strip and weigh myself again, I'm still virtually the same weight, and then I catch sight of my fully naked body, stomach distended with an assortment of unnecessary binge food, my waist has disappeared and I swear I can see another layer of cellulite forming before my very eyes. That does it. I go and get on slob clothes and cancel going out. I decide to stay in and 'make a night of it', ready to start again tomorrow. Videos and sad music at the ready and over the course of the next few hours, I gradually complete the classic 'major' binge by forcing down the following:

- Three big glasses of Bailey's with ice.

- Entire contents of a 24hr mini-mart, bought in midst of frantic binge-mode containing the following:

- Marshmallow biscuits - four and a half of a pack of six.

- Viennese whirls - another favourite - ate three of six - everyone more difficult to stomach than the last.

- Honey roast peanuts - the type I usually avoid because they're too high in calories.

- Smoked mackerel - I usually avoid this when I'm on a counting the fat diet - decided to take advantage of the binge and have one.

Now I feel really sick.

- Crusty rolls and butter - hoping for sponge-like effect to soak up the fat.

- Two tomatoes and four slices of cucumber - a token gesture, which fails dismally to make me feel better.

- Still room for another Twix and three more Bounty bars.

What Does Your Binge Look Like?

Have you got binge-paralysis now, just thinking about it? It's ok, you're not there yet. You can be if you want to be, or maybe this time you could just eat the food on condition you enjoy it, and when it stops being enjoyable, you can leave it till later. How do you usually feel at the end of it? When is enough enough? When you go to sleep? And even then you wake up just to get a few more calories down you whilst it's still technically' yesterday'. With me a binge used to be less a case of 'in for a penny, in for a pound', and more 'in for a penny, in for a limited edition, solid 24 carat gold sovereign, set with diamond inlay, signed certificate of authenticity and leather gift box'. Extreme to the max. Rarely done by halves, unless a miracle or distraction occurred. I always viewed my binge as if it would be positively the last time. In fact, this was obligatory in order to accept the binge would happen - it had to be the last time-ever. It always made me feel worthless, and confirmed my suspicions that my whole life would be permanently on hold until I could get this weight thing sorted out. And it was all my body's fault, and it just couldn't be trusted.

Record your feelings if you feel like. This helps you to anchor this rotten feeling at the start of a binge instead of to the end. What's it feel like afterwards? How much do you hate yourself? What's going to be postponed yet again through having binged and therefore losing a day's dieting? See with me, it used to be like this, my friend Marion reminded me of it when we sat chatting about binging the other day.

Anatomy of a Binge.

At the start of a binge, you get that sheer relief. When you get up to go to the kitchen knowing you're on your way to giving in and 'treating yourself'. You've accepted that the diet ends again now, and you just need that treat in your body. You can justify it somehow. Maybe it'll be just the one snack, though, this time.

Then again maybe not. The first taste is sheer relief. It's heaven. Welcome back old friend. The chocolate you denied yourself is now rightfully yours once more. And the pleasure is extreme. Not only pleasure that you're eating the food, but pleasure that you're doing what you want instead of adhering to someone else's diet and rules. "I'll show them." Maybe it doesn't start out to be a major binge, but the pattern is hard to break, and off you go again, into the dreaded... Binge Funnel. And when it starts to suck you down, my God is it powerful, and you just have to go with it because it's a well-trodden pathway. You're on auto pilot, your body and mind knows where to go, and you are helpless in its grasp. Whatever else you can't do in your life right now, you certainly know how to have a good binge. It's the certainty and significance of it all. You know where you are with a binge. You're in control whilst deliciously out of control. Deeper and deeper into the binge funnel till there's nothing but black and no turning back, no stopping, no passing go or collecting two hundred pounds worth of binge-food.

Then it ceases to be about having food. It's stopped being about the pleasure of eating. After a while, only the 'taste-on-the-tongue' pleasure, and the, 'saying yes, not no' pleasure remains. After that it becomes about self-flagellation. Beating yourself up and punishing yourself because you're such a bad person. You're repulsive, no wonder boys don't want you or find you attractive. Or no wonder you don't get that job you want, or whatever, ad infinitum. You deserve to feel like shit. So eat this, and this, and that. Take that, and that. Force it down. Make yourself feel sick, you deserve to. Maybe you'll get round to throwing it up afterwards. Maybe not. Sure as hell you'll be back on the diet/ famine - an even stricter one than before - as soon as day breaks tomorrow.

It's All in the Brain.

From then on it's all about a battle in your brain - if you can't control yourself enough not to eat what you should, you can sure as hell prove you're in control by eating what you shouldn't, big time, and then it becomes a matter of repeating old patterns, sticking with your identity. It's a well-trodden path, remember? And then punishing yourself for eating too much by, well, eating even more. Till you make yourself feel ill. Really, really ill. Isn't it amazing in this modern world when there's so much that's wrong out there already, and so much we're capable of, that so many perfectly-normal-in-most-other-ways adult females - and some males - can bring on this self-inflicted misery? Whether it's food or cigarettes, or drugs, or drink, or sheer depression, it's all a variation on a theme- things that we bring about through what goes on in our head. So if we create it in our head, we have to end it in our head. Unless there's a physiological reason or deficiency in our bodies (see Julia Ross' book The Diet Cure, and your own doctor), then we are all capable of ending it, and just like the beginning, the end has to start in our heads.

And this book may be the very first step.

It's not impossible to stop it. If you think it is impossible, and that you have to keep bingeing in exactly the same way, even if it's your own unique way, with your own conditions, then it's because you choose not to stop it. Maybe it fulfils some need in you like certainty, variety or perhaps, significance, ie, it's the closest you might feel to love at the moment, connection with yourself and a type of behaviour you know very well. There may even be a little bit of growth, as you expand the amount you can consume at one sitting, and even some contribution, to your own conviction that you truly are a bad person incapable of reforming. Six human needs, according to Tony Robbins, remember?[(21)] And if the diet/binge situation suits you because having those needs fulfilled is more important than breaking free, then imprisoned you will stay.

The only thing you can do is just stop complaining about it! Develop a new set of beliefs and tell yourself what you're doing your regular bingeing and the rules you have about the way you do it - is ok, it's just part of you. But then so is being fat. And for many people being what you'd call 'fat' is actually ok, remember. So what's it to be - you decide. Just stop whingeing about it. You make the choices, you bear the consequences.

Time to change?

Yes, we can opt to keep thinking the same thoughts the same way with the same outcome every single day of the year for the rest of our lives if we want. If that's what you want, then that's your choice too, and it makes you no different from the countless other non-extraordinary people who can't break free from their rules either. It's up to you. It's all a matter of making choices. But I'm not talking about sheer willpower here. No-one is more against the whole idea of sheer willpower being the only thing you need to overcome any urge your body sends to your mind, or any urge your mind sends your body. Willpower's fine, but it's not the be all and end all. It's not the whole story. The same people who stick to diets compulsively their whole lives through are often the same sort of people who do everything in their lives in the same rigid, strict way. That's not most of us. What we need to do is be sensible - go back to basics, back to nature. We need to listen to our bodies. Our bodies have an important role to play in the way we live our lives, and half the trouble we've got ourselves into is because we started over-riding these important body signals in the first place. So

I'm not saying overcome your over eating and bingeing urge by beating yourself up saying it's all about self-control, and that you're weak if you don't manage to stick to a diet/ famine regimentally. I'm saying do it the natural way - the way the body was intended to be - a two way street of communication. And this means, be kind to yourself. If you're forcing your body to overeat, especially to binge level, then you're just doing a variation of the macho willpower thing and overriding your body's important signals surrounding eating, instead of listening to the subtle nuances it gives out when it's time to stop, or time to sleep, or time to exercise, or rest and so on. We just need to re-learn the language. But step by step, with the natural approach.

So the next step now in binge management would be to think about some of these signals, listen, and communicate with your body. First and foremost, is it time to eat yet? **Preferably wait till you're really hungry.** This goes without saying as a part of true Food Freedom, and if you're just browsing through and this is the first bit of this book that you're reading, then do look up the relevant section about being truly body hungry before you decide when to eat. Then you can go to the next step of **Food Freedom** which is binge-management, and the question of what.

Now it's time to begin.

Staying on the rim of the binge funnel. Instead of being sucked downwards in a never-ending spiral, what I'm hoping to help you with, is to accept that you need to change your pattern at this crucial point, before it's too late and you're too far into the binge to be able to break free. It's freedom of a more advanced kind to be able to step out of the box and take yourself somewhere else when in a binge frame of mind. Believe me, the liberation you'll feel will be enormous, the sort of feeling you get when you step on the scales and find out you've lost a pound or two when you haven't really even been trying. A good feeling. Something new! Be adventurous at this point in your life - when all else has let you down - it's not your inability to stick at it that's made it fail for you, believe me. It's the diet's fault not yours. Everyone else is going to stay stuck in the binge funnel for the rest of their lives, but you can be the one that breaks free, ok? You've got the rest of your life to go back to the same behaviour, so for now, just give this a try. Let me be your success coach, and help you through this period in your life, but do it all in your own time, in a way that feels right, and works for you, or don't do it at all. Ok? And then in the future at some stage, you'll look back at the period you've just been going through - however long it is - and it'll be like some distant memory. So assuming you're up for it, you're going to step up and take your life to its next level, and with the initial help of binge management, get rid of this demon thing that keeps messing with your head and consequently with your body. So what's next? Well, if you're dieting, and you're still convinced that's the only way to lose weight, but the diet starts tomorrow, here's what to do about the choice of food to eat now.

Think about what you really feel like most.

Of course, there's much more about these topics in the other parts of the book, and they're there for you when you're ready, but in a nutshell, for the desperate person on-the-verge-of-a-binge, here's what you do.

Become a food detective.

Go and get all the foods in front of you. All the foods you'd normally force down you, in this binge you're about to have. I'm not saying you have to eat the lot, and I'm certainly not saying you can't. I'm not saying you have to now count what's in each of them and limit yourself, by calories or fat grams or carbs and so on, exercising yet more deprivation and control before changing your mind and eating the lot anyway. No, don't count anything, and if you find you still want the lot, you are being given full permission to eat every single last bit. As usual. But since you're off the diet anyway, use this occasion as an important experiment with Food Freedom. I'll talk you through it. So off you go. Go and get all the binge foods. Don't underestimate it either. I want you to get every single type of food you'd normally eat. If they need preparation, just bring them as they are - still boxed if there's a picture on the box. That'll work almost as well. If it's just a pile of ingredients, it may not give you the right feedback, so do whatever you'd normally need to do with the food before you eat it. Unless you'd normally eat ingredients! In which case, bring them on! Now, with them all in front of you, I want you to look at each one, and work out which appeals to you most.

Virtual dining.

This is one of the most important steps. Think about it. Feel it.

If you want, do some Virtual Dining. To help you make your choices by imagining the flavour in your mouth, and what it feels like afterwards, thereby helping you to know which is the best one for you right now.

If you're truly body-hungry at this point, some things will probably shout out at you more than others. If you've decided to try it too early and you're not hungry enough, or maybe you've just had dinner, do it now anyway, and just pay more attention to the signals, then try to be hungry enough next time. Maybe tasting a little of each will help - the one your body needs most will taste the best. Some people will have laid out foods with a wide cross-section of flavours - savoury, salty, bitter, sweet and different textures - crispy, bland, crunchy, or chewy. Other people may just have a tray/table or floor full of variations on a theme, for example chocolate. If that's your decision this time, then fine. Another time see if you can bring in a bit more choice, as you'll notice the markedly different reactions your body has to the different types of food. Same thing if you're hungry - it'll make for better choices, and a better experiment.

Which shouts at you the most?

That's the one to eat first. And the others in descending order of appeal. Forget balance. Forget previous patterns. For example, you always have the stir fry and vegetables first in an effort to fill yourself up so you're not hungry any more. Or you always have the steamed broccoli to feel like you're getting an even mixture and at least some goodness, or, you always binge on chocolate, so that's what you always have. Maybe chocolate isn't the thing that's jumping out at you this time. Perhaps it's the roast potato or the tuna soaked in olive oil.

Letting your body decide may be the turning point you've always longed for.

Tell you why. When I first started doing Food Freedom, one of the most amazing effects it had, pretty early on, was removing the 'secret treasure factor', from bad foods.

The secret treasure factor.

You know what I mean? Every 'bad' food is like a precious booty you treat it like it's treasure, covet it, always want it even at inappropriate times, hoard it, hide it, want it in times of stress, use it as a comforter. Damn it, just owning it makes you feel better. You take it away on holiday with you or to an overnight stay just so you'll be prepared and just in case you feel you're going to need an emergency supply. But you often don't let anyone know about it. Because it's yours - your secret - your treasure.

So in a binge, you purely seek treasure, and load up on it, get as much as you can of it, in order to stock up and help battle the deprivation just around the corner. **But remove the treasure factor and those foods aren't quite so important in your life any more.** And what happens when we can have something we want, without telling ourselves, 'no' anymore? What happens when there's no restriction on something we've always deprived ourselves of? Well, you'll find out if you follow this process. But my reaction was, all of a sudden, "do I really want it then?" The answer came back more and more often, "no." Or, crucially in a binge, not so much of it then. How many times have I started a little 'off the wagon' session, intending it to be just that, a little session, and ended up having yet another Last Supper? You've done it too, huh? Well, if you can Freedom Eat your way through a binge, you never know, you may find you like the idea of it so much that you want to carryon doing it this new way instead of ever going back to a deprivation diet again. If it doesn't work permanently then what's the point? Would you keep going back to the same garage to get the same repair done if the car still kept reverting to the old problem every time? If even a shred of you says, 'absolutely not,' then please do listen carefully to the next bit - this is where Food Freedom gets really clever.

Do nothing else at all whilst eating the food. Give each mouthful your total attention.

End of story. No preparing the next bite. No reading the paper at the same time, just, take a bite, chew it, attend it, swallow it, You'll notice and remember every mouthful instead of suddenly finding all the sandwich has gone but you don't recall eating it, but no-one else has done so, so it must be you. It's hard initially if you're conditioned to read/watch TV/drive/talk or cry at the same time. But it's only a learned behaviour. It really doesn't have to be part of your identity. Ever wanted to be someone else? Well it starts right here. How can you get used to the idea of being this slimmer person if you can't even adapt a bit right now, especially when it means you can sit and really enjoy each bite of food? Believe me, try it a few times, and you'll enjoy it, get used to it before too long, and find it a comforting part of the whole eating process, and guess what? It's the way we were supposed to do it! See the other parts of the book about this topic for more details.

Listen for satisfied.

Now comes the really clever bit. If you can stop when your body has had enough food, sufficient food for the time being even during a binge, look for the point when the taste changes and the flavour diminishes. If you can let yourself wait a bit before eating some more, and if you can tryout the unusual notion that you don't have to make it into a Last Supper, then you'll be giving yourself a handful of true freedom. And that's not to be underestimated. Elsewhere in this book I'll be explaining more about how to tell if you're satisfied - an important distinction from 'full'. But basically, you should feel light and comfortable, energetic not lethargic, and you shouldn't be able to feel the food in your stomach, and you should have eaten maybe a portion of food no bigger roughly than a fist, and the 'drop dead gorgeous' taste will have dissipated. For me the biggest sign is that my body breathes a deep abdominal breath, as if to say, "haaahhh, that's better, thank you, I needed that, now I'm done." I generally take a mouthful or two more, and that's it.

If you can't seem to stop at this point, keep telling yourself that all this food is yours, no-one's saying you can't have it, just wait a little while till you're hungry again and you can have as much more of it as you want at that time too. Or something else that's not on the pile. Or forget the lot and go out for a salad. Or lose interest in it all because it's no longer out of bounds. Or find something more interesting to do instead, which may go some way to satisfying the real craving inside you. It's often not food we want, at times like this. It just feels like food-hunger, because we've always used food as the answer to every craving we've had all our lives. Or we've learned to later on. Habit again, see? But we don't have to be sheep and follow everyone else all the time. What about starting to discover what it is you really want right now. Is it hunger, really? If several mouthfuls of sweets didn't do it, and the same 'hunger' comes right back, then it's not hunger for food.

Fine if you decide to feed it with food anyway. You would have gone ahead and had a huge binge anyway, so it makes no odds if you do the same old thing again now. It's up to you. If you want to eat more right now, do it. But what if this can be the beginning of finding out what your body's really telling you? What if this can be the start of a beautiful friendship? A wonderful partnership? Rather than you hating it and not being able to trust it - you think.

Think about what your body's been feeling all this time? "Silly brain - keeps over-riding my signals. Told it time after time I don't want any more to eat right now. I didn't want those chips that time and I didn't need a potato right now - so I made it taste like cardboard. Why did my brain make me eat it when it didn't taste great, and the chicken, peas and gravy was what I really wanted, and some water. Still I'll be there for you, brain. When the rain starts to pour. I'll be here for you. Like I've been here before. I'll be here for you. If you'd only be there for me too ... "

Or else, quit the binge - for a while at least - and go and find something that really fulfils your need. At one point I realised it was just a need to be held in my husband's arms. I love being hugged. It fulfils some physiological need in me. I ache when I haven't been hugged for a while. Sometimes I need a hug more than others. When I've gone without a man in my life - the time I'm thinking of is nearly a year without a boyfriend, and I yearned so badly for someone, so I fed the yearning with food for ten months solid. And ended up thirteen and a half stone. There aren't many times I've been that weight in my life - and not pregnant. **So thank God now for Food Freedom. Because becoming body aware means I can recognise the signals that my body sends me and know that food, although a fleeting consolation, is not always the right answer.** So go and find out what is and read the other sections of this book for more ideas.

Then become a food detective once more. You did it at the start to help decide what to eat, now do it after the food's in your body to help make your choices the right ones for you and your body long term. No-one's saying that with Food Freedom, you have an excuse for a perpetual binge. If you're not stopping at satisfied, and you're over-filling your 'gas tank', then the petrol is going to spill out of the fuel tank and into the storage area which are your hips and thighs and stomach and all the other places where your body stores its excess fat. If you eat too much, you'll still feel lethargic afterwards. Your body is communicating with you, so listen, and more importantly, respond. If you can work out which part of the meal you just ate gave you wind, or a headache, or made you feel rather short of breath, or tired a few hours later, or whatever, then experiment. In true Sherlock Holmes fashion, work out how you can alter it next time. Have it with water, have the protein without the carb, have no mayonnaise, have brown instead of white, have more olive oil and start making it acceptable for your body.

If your body likes what you're giving it, it will let you know. If it doesn't, it will let you know.

And if we can sort out the 'good for me' from the 'not so good for me in that combination.' It will save you masses of time in the future. Instead of trying all the different diet and eating plans under the sun, in the vain hope that a food plan designed for the masses can possibly meet all your personal requirements and also in the vain hope of finding one that may be custom-built just for your body. Instead, you can work out your own, by being your very own food detective. Then at least you'll be aware of the effect of your choices on your body, even if you don't particularly like the aftereffects.

And so with a binge, try using Food Freedom Binge Management to help cope the next time you feel a binge coming on.

And one day, when you're through with diets, because you realise that they're only a self-imposed famine to which your body has to react to save itself from starving, by lowering your metabolism and thereby the amount of food you can consume without putting on weight, then you'll be ready to become a fully-fledged Freedom Eater and live your life with Food Freedom, instead of in Food Prison.

And finally ...

So that's it in a nutshell then. Food Freedom can help dieters through a binge as well as every other person escape from their own particular food prison. The Freedom Eating girls are my saviours when it comes to 'falling off the path'. Don't think it's an overnight transformation - it's a 'getting to know yourself again' process, and that takes time. But it's bloody enjoyable. What? When every meal is a pleasure - a true pleasure not a forbidden one - because every morsel is eaten in a state when your body is ready for it, when you really are body hungry. It's concentrated on, given your total attention and enjoyed, as food should be. You stop when the flavour of the food diminishes because your body's had enough so it decreases the tumultuous enjoyment of each successive mouthful, and that tells you that you're satisfied. Therefore you stop before you get to feeling full - overloaded, sick, heavy, lethargic, uncomfortable. For those reasons, every meal is total pleasure, never a chore or a punishment or something to be feared. Then you're following it up with an awareness process which helps you pick up yet more signals from your own physiology which helps you refine your choice-making next time round, helping you be a food detective and to communicate with your body in an ever-more sophisticated way. Eventually you should be able to intuitively feel in advance what your body will feel like for every extra ounce of cereal you pour into the bowl. You'll just know how much you need. And that means one big happy bunny where food's concerned, rather than being a pain-in-the-neck, same-as-everyone-else, completely un-extraordinary, weak-and-feeble, no willpower, disgusting-useless-good-for-nothing, or substitute other alternatives you usually use about yourself on a regular basis, every time you break the latest diet/famine.

That's all it comes down to, you know. It's all just a matter of unlearning the rules that have brought us to where we are now on the food cycle. Go back to basics. Break out of prison. Food prison.

And the next time you feel like bingeing again, pick up this book once more, and try it over again. The more opportunities you give yourself to do it, the easier and more natural it will be. So don't worry that you 'can't trust yourself' to do Food Freedom straight away. Just do whatever you feel you should be doing - whatever's right for you - diet, whatever. And use this book like a faithful friend in times of trouble. The one who will hold your hand and say, "it's ok" even through the toughest food-crisis, because this method is all about the long-term, not the quick-fixes, or the rules and regulations.

You've had enough control and deprivation in your life. Now try a little freedom.

Footnote

When you first find out about a system like this, you may get all fired up and enthusiastic - and well you should be - it's a solid common sense system, with its basis firmly in nature. But I want to say a few things now, as food for thought. **It won't work if you don't do it.** Someone once said to me, "Food Freedom stopped working for me." Why? Because she stopped using it, and had gone back to dieting. If that's your choice too, then fine. But re-read the book if you start to lose your way. They say we should do something a good twenty times or for a good four weeks, before we can get into the habit of it. The same is true of Food Freedom. But once you do learn it, my God is it a turn around in your life and if I can do it, *believe me* you can too.

Since changing my life with Food Freedom, I've actually been keeping the weight off. And if you knew what I've been through in the last three years, that's an amazing feat. And yes, sure I've had little lapses into a little comfort eating, but they're little ones and they're soon rectified. In fact what's happened to me in the last year alone (2001) would have definitely made me comfort eat my way to at least an extra stone and a half, had I not had this system to rely on and get me back on the straight and narrow.

But that's a story for another book! For now, you know enough to get you going on one of the most amazing life-changing systems I've ever known. And in more than seven years of shopping telly, I've seen a lot of systems!

Ask yourself how many people you know who've gained a lot of weight, lost it and actually kept it off for more than a year. Well now you know one more - me. And it's all so easy now. And it can be for you too - seriously - you just have to learn to trust yourself. Trust your body's messages, maybe for the first time ever. If you don't try, you'll never know - and what have you got to lose? Will it be another ten binges before you decide to give it a go? Or are you going to take the plunge right now. Go on, go on, go on, go on. Need more insights? Let me help you.

Let me give you a picture of what it can be like for me nowadays, as a food prison escapee ...

This weekend, I went to a reunion of my Piccadilly Radio colleagues after fifteen years. Stressful? Absolutely. The old me would have binged all the way there in the car, then made sure I bagged myself a good plate full of the buffet, including dessert and coffee. Then having survived the evening, I'd have gone back to the hotel, armed with a bag of goodies for a solo binge, which I'd have made sure included half the mini bar snacks, and all the coffees, hot chocolate and biscuits on the tea tray in the room too. Then in the morning, I'd have made sure I got up and had the breakfast I'd paid for, even if it meant having a cooked breakfast I didn't really feel like, and balanced it out with some fruit and yoghurt just because it was there. Oh, and a token bit of jam on toast into the bargain. And taken what I could with me, including the mini marmalade, even though it was actually apricot jam and would sit in the cupboard at home for two years.

That was the old me. Know what the new Food Freedom - liberated me did? Because I was actually ready to eat on the M6 when I stopped for petrol on the way up to Manchester, I got a chicken burger and onion rings - no fries, I didn't feel like them. But I did feel like a bit of Twix, and that's what I had - the rest of it I put in the glove box for another time, and when I got to the party, I still wasn't hungry, so I didn't have anything. I really, genuinely didn't want it. Nor the breakfast the next morning. Just an orange juice with my friend Diane who popped by for a coffee before I headed back south to the kids. Another time, I would've been at Sainsbury's supermarket by teatime, but now, and because I eat late, myself, I can have a coffee, with a big glass of water, and be quite happy just sitting there with the kids whilst they eat their dinner in a restaurant. Amazing. The old me would have instinctively chosen to eat a meal... well just because.

And last Christmas, I can't tell you how great it was. The year before was the first Christmas I hadn't put on weight. I've avoided putting on a few pounds as a result of succumbing to scarcity fever that I always used to believe was an intrinsic part of the festive season, for two successive Christmases. It's finally working.

I truly am a new me.

I do try to contemplate the healthy option whenever I can, and to be honest, having complete freedom to choose any food means I regularly take the healthy option, naturally. Whilst Food Freedom advocates having anything you really want - no food is off bounds. We all know that healthier is better. But if you can break free from food prison, guess what? Your body will know what to choose healthily anyway. This system should get you to the point of being able to desire the healthier options without needing to check in with your brain. It's just that if you're in a position of being screwed up as a result of so many years of deprivation and control. Or if you beat yourself up regularly about making the wrong food choices, then you need to let go totally, and maybe even go through a brief 'eating crap' stage, before you can start truly meeting your body's needs to listening to it.

So don't think you can use this book as an excuse to eat only rubbish for ever more. If you do, you aren't doing Food Freedom. Just keep the book and its contents for when you're totally ready for it.

As your body adapts to its new found freedom, and you let go of the old restrictive behaviours, all kinds of weird things may happen including initial up and down fluctuations in weight and strange reactions from friends and family. Just acknowledge, let go, learn and move on. If it feels good, then do it, do it right, and you will definitely start feeling good - better than you have done in years!

In which case, I'd love to hear about it! There are some stories, included in this book, from some lovely people who were kind enough to write to me in the past. Please see the details at the end of this book, on ways not only to contact me via the website, but also to find out about other products, and further reading mentioned in this book, or how you can get hold of the associated audio cassette programme.

For now remember that if it feels good, it's probably doing you good, and every big change starts with the tiniest baby step, so make one today. Good luck with breaking free from food prison forever.

Debbie

The Key Points to Food Freedom

1- Only eat when you're physically hungry.

2- Only eat till you're satisfied, not till you're full.

3- Give the food your full attention.

4- Think about what your body really needs, not what your brain really wants.

5- You can do this even if you're on a diet.

6- If you want something 'bad', go ahead and eat it. Or maybe if during one meal, you end up overeating slightly, just don't beat yourself up about it afterwards.

7 - Be an observer, not a judge.

8- Don't set yourself up to fail by having too many rules. Forget every old rule surrounding food.

9- Listen to how your body responds to the food in your stomach and learn how to make a good match. Learn to trust your body.

10- Don't forget the water thing.

11- Keep listening.

12- Accept whatever shape and weight your body wants to be.

13- Don't let others, or your own thoughts, get you down.

14- Stand guard at the door of your mind.

Testimonials - 1999 - 2002

Dear Debbie,

I bought the Freedom Eating Plan in September 2000 and I'm so grateful that I did. At that point in my life I had been bulimic for eighteen years and was more and more desperate to be 'normal'. I would look at my three children and feel jealous that they could eat anything they liked and I couldn't at the age of thirty one. I couldn't face the thought of never eating the things I wanted or having to eat diet versions for the rest of my life. When I read the book, I alternated between crying and shouting, "yes that's me". I felt as though a great weight had lifted from me. I have never been very overweight (due, I suppose to the bulimia). But I was chubby. Since September it has melted away and I have lost approximately a stone and I feel normal. Better yet I have eaten foods I thought I was not 'allowed'. My husband has noticed the weight difference and the personality difference. I am no longer obsessed by food. I buy lovely delicious food without guilt and with complete enjoyment. Please pass my thanks to the girls for this gift of common sense.

Yours sincerely.

Jane

Dear Debbie,

I watched your programme and was moved to write to you. I bought the Freedom Eating Book and tape at its original launch. I was at an all time low. I was being treated for very severe depression and was at home feeling very sorry for myself I hate to confess but I was wearing size a 18 and hated my body. I felt as if everything was out to get me. The excitement and enthusiasm from Shawn and Vikki caught my attention so I gave it a go'. I can honestly say that my life has been turned around. I have gone down to a size 14 and I feel great. My depression has gone. I get compliments and praise for all my hard work. I feel like a fraud because it was so easy. I just wish I had discovered Freedom Eating ten years ago. My only problem is what to do with the dozens of clothes that just swim on me.

Laura

Dear Debbie,

Hi. I hope this letter finds you in good health. I had to write to you. I do hope you don't mind. My children are a similar age to yours (boy and girl - Chris & Laura) and my weight has been a nightmare since I was first pregnant. When I booked into the hospital I was ten stone. Seven months later I was nearly sixteen stone and I'd had the baby. I have tried everything. I even worked for a national slimming organisation at one point and when I heard that Vicki Hansen had worked for Weight Watchers I realised how similar we were. Over the last thirteen years I've been nine stone and sixteen stone and everywhere in between. I just couldn't get a handle on it. I am in control over everything else in my life and I couldn't understand why food should be such a problem. I purchased 'The Seven Secrets Slim People' in 1999. I read it over and over but I wasn't convinced. I've spent so long either being totally strict and calorie counting or bingeing either on a diet or off it that I couldn't believe it would work especially for me 5'5" and 15 stone. I was sure I was a complete no hoper. However, when you had the Freedom eating segment, I was ready to give it a go. What a revelation. I've lost four pounds this week but much better than that, I am back in control of me. I cannot thank you enough for bringing this to me I really do think it's life changing.

Name supplied

Dear Debbie.

I have always been a couple of stones overweight for as long as I can remember. Then about eight years ago I used slimming pills to get from twelve stone to 8 st 13 lbs. However I did not address the real problem of my obsession with food and needless to say the weight came back and I just kept getting bigger. I'm thirty one years old and weigh 20 stone 9 lbs. Since I bought the Seven Secrets package, I have to say I really feel cured of all the food related problems in my life. This way of looking at eating has done more for me than any diet, doctor or counsellor that I have sought help from before. I have lost nearly four stone since I had my baby last August. I am so happy and so grateful not to feel like I am a freak of nature or a hopeless failure because I couldn't diet properly. Now I am looking forward to a free and happy future, I discovered that I smothered feelings under food and now I am learning to deal with what my spirit is hungry for. As suggested in the original Seven Secrets and the Powerplus pack (which is also fantastic) I have decided to study for qualifications that will get me a job that I will enjoy and I am at last finding ways of venting my stress and anger. Instead of eating myself to death, I feel like a worthwhile normal person. This new feeling of self-esteem and self-confidence is priceless.

With love, thanks and best wishes
Nina

Dear Debbie,

My reason for trying Freedom Eating was that at the time I was in an unsatisfying relationship, and I realise now that I was overeating as a way of convincing myself that everything was ok. The package does take a lot of getting used to... but more importantly I haven't been on the scales for six months and haven't put on any weight over Christmas for the first time that I can remember. I exercise quite frequently which I enjoy and I've gone down from a size 16 to a 14. People have even commented that I look like I've lost weight. I know I still have a long way to go yet but the best thing about the whole process is that there is no time limit and that I feel I have some free-will over my life again.

Thank you for all your help.

Dyane

The above testimonials were received by the author, in connection with the promotion of the Freedom Eating concept, as it appears in The Seven Secrets of Slim People *by V.Hansen and J.Goodman while the author was a presenter on QVC, and afterwards, spanning 1999-2001*

Appendix - References

1. Keys, A. ,Brozek, J., Henschel,A., Mickelsen, O.,Taylor,H.L.(l950) The Biology of Human Starvation,Minneapolis:University of Minnesota Press.

2.6.8. Freedom Eating -Program One- (1997), *The Seven Secrets of Slim People, audio cassettes.*

3. T, Robbins, *Personal Power 2*.(1996), audio cassettes and CD sets and www.robbins.com Robbins Research International Inc.

4.19. W. Dyers Erroneous Zones, (1988),Time Warner Paperbacks.

5. V. Hansen and S. Goodman, The Seven Secrets of Slim People (1997), Hay House Inc. USA

7. Pearson,L. The Psychologist's Eat-Anything Diet,(1993) Peter H 179 Publishers, p 250.

9. T. Robbins, *Unleash the Power Within Weekends*,London Arena July 2001.

10. T. Robbins, *Power to Influence Seminars,* London, Nov 2001.

11. Sims, EAH., Goldman, R., Gluck, C. Horton, E.S Kelleher, P.,& Rowe, D.(1968). *Experimental Obesity in Man*. Transcript of the Association of American Physicians, 81, 153.

12. Bennet, W. and Gurin, J.(1982) The Dieter's Dilemma: Eating Less and Weighing More, New York:Basic Books.

13. Louise Hay and Bernie Siegel, *You Can Heal Your Life*, Audio Cassettes,(l996), Hay house inc. London Hodder Headline Audio Books.
14.17. www.TonyRobbins.com

15.19. Wayne Dyer, *Pulling your Own Strings*, (1990) Arrow.

16. Magical Body, Magical Mind, CD set, Deepak Chopra. Nightingale Conant

18. www.pentawater.com. C.2001

20. S. Gawain, *Creative Visualisations*,(1998) audio cassettes. Bantam Press.

21. T. Robbins, *Personal Power 2*, (1996) Audio cassette and CD set, Robbins Research International

Further reading & Support Groups Online

- V. Hansen and J. Goodman, The Seven Secrets of Slim People (1997), Hay House Inc. USA

- B. Schwarz, Diets Don't Work, (1995) Breakthrough Publishing.

- Julia Ross, The Diet Cure, (2001), Penguin Press.

This book was originally published in 2001 by Sahara Publishing.
Some of the references are out of date in 2014.
If there is any aspect of this information you would like to clarify, see below on how to contact author.

Debbie Flint returned to QVC the Shopping Channel in 2009.
Her weekly blog can be found at http://blogs.qvcuk.com/debbie_flint/

If you like this book, get in touch and let her know.

SUPPORT

Join the Facebook group 'Till the Fat Lady Slims' –

https://www.facebook.com/groups/TTFLS/

Bonus Material

Please visit my website for news of how to get your free bonus audio material supporting this book:

.....Podcasts covering even more aspects of Freedom Eating, including the full conversation with ex-slimming club leader Linda Bignell.

.... A relaxation track to further enhance your journey out of Food Prison (coming January 2015.)

EXTRA MATERIAL – can be found on my website

www.debbieflint.co.uk/TTFLS

Where prompted, please use bonus code TTFLS20140929

BONUS EXCLUSIVE MATERIAL for readers of this book –

www.debbieflint.co.uk/BONUS

enter password code TTFLSQVC2015

PLUS .... The newest testimonials from the Facebook group 'TTFLS'

Or add your own testimonials by emailing debbie@debbieflint.com

Also available – Debbie's fiction

(eBook or paperback)

'Diary of a Wannabe Shopping Channel Presenter' - Bridget Jones meets Alan Partridge meets Eddie Murphy in Holy Man the movie in this humorous romp, written in journal style.

'When Dreams Return' - a spooky short story with a twist.

'Valentine's Surprise' - a gentle romance to warm your heart, a short story for a rainy day - it's never too late to find your Sir Lancelot.

'The Hawaiian Trilogy' – Sadie Turner and Helen Parker are sisters facing the biggest decisions of their lives. In Hawaiian Escape we go from Tuscany to New York in a race to win a life-changing competition. In Hawaiian Affair, we follow Sadie's trip to Hawaii via a case of mistaken identity on a luxury yacht in Monaco. And in Hawaiian Retreat, Helen's story unfolds, taking her to a breath-taking climax for Try it For the First Time Club, featuring exciting events in Tibet, Thailand and Italy. Will the sisters find their true loves or will they choose business over pleasure?

UPDATES – KEEP IN TOUCH

For the latest updates on Debbie Flint's work, a free steamy download, and news of sequels, prequels, and more romance, visit www.debbieflint.com to sign up for the regular newsletter alerts - be the first to find out about brand new titles.

Twitter - @debbieflint

Or www.facebook.com/DebbieFlintQVCUK

Published by flintproductions